The Bare Facts of
Systemic Pathology

The Bare Facts of Systemic Pathology

Joseph A. Sisson, M.D.

Professor of Pathology
Creighton University
School of Medicine; Director, Creighton University
School of Medical Technology,
Omaha, Nebraska

SECOND EDITION

*Illustrated by Robert Goad, and by the Graphic Arts Section, Creighton University
Biomedical Communications*

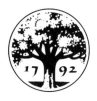

J. B. Lippincott Company
Philadelphia   Toronto

ISBN 0–397–52085–9

Library of Congress Catalog Card Number 78–478

Printed in the United States of America

3 5 6 4

Library of Congress Cataloging in Publication Data

Sisson, Joseph A
    The bare facts of systemic pathology.

    Includes index.
    1. Pathology—Outlines, syllabi, etc. I. Title.
    [DNLM: 1. Pathology—Outlines, QZ18 S623ba]
    RB111S47   1978   616.07   78–478
    ISBN 0–397–52085–9

To Pauline

Preface

This completely revised and updated edition of *The Bare Facts of Systemic Pathology* presents in succinct, synoptic, modular form the salient features of pathologic conditions as they affect the organ systems. To achieve this goal, tables, lists, side-by-side comparisons and brief passages of "pathologic prose" are used as appropriate. In this second edition I have kept the original "Bare Facts" approach intact as much as possible, adding only what seems new and significant and deleting what is no longer considered true or relevant.

Traditionally, this book has been most useful to medical students taking courses in pathology and preparing clinical presentations during the last 2 years of medical school. Students and physicians preparing for National Boards (parts I and II), have also found this book very helpful. Recently, many new physicians have told me that this book is an excellent review in preparation for taking the FLEX examination, especially for the Clinical Sciences and Clinical Competence portions.

With its companion volumes, *The Bare Facts of General Pathology* and *The Handbook of Clinical Pathology,* this book forms a complete modular method or system for rapidly acquiring knowledge of pathology needed by the modern practicing physician. Together these volumes cover the range of topics traditionally confronting the medical school course in pathology as well as the clinical application of this knowledge, including the use of laboratory tests in the clinical disciplines such as Surgery, Medicine, Obstetrics, Gynecology and Pediatrics.

Joseph A. Sisson, M.D.

Acknowledgments

For the preparation of the second edition of *The Bare Facts of Systemic Pathology,* I would like to acknowledge the help of Miss Pauline Jadick, who has been with the "Bare Facts" since its inception. I would also like to thank my secretary, Miss Rita Christensen, for her stenographic assistance.

Joseph A. Sisson, M.D.

Contents

Abbreviations Used in This Text

ABBREVIATION	TERM	ABBREVIATION	TERM
ACTH	Adrenocorticotropic hormone	CVA	Cerebrovascular accident (stroke); costovertebra angle
ADH	Antidiuretic hormone		
AFIP	Armed Forces Institute of Pathology	DDD	para Dichlorodiphenyl-dichloroethane
A/G	Albumin globulin ratio	DIP	Desquamative interstitial pneumonitis
AGBM	Antiglomerular basement membrane	DNA	Deoxyribonucleic acid
AGBMA	Antiglomerular basement membrane antibody	Dx	Diagnosis
		EEE	Eastern equine encephalitis
ASD	Atrial septal defect	EKG	Electrocardiogram
ATA	Antithyroid antibody	EM	Electron micrograph, electron microscopic
AUM	Asymmetric unit membrane	EOM	Extraocular muscles
AV	Atrioventricular node or valve	EPI	Anatomic: above Clinical: isomeric to a reference compound
BCH	Basal cell hyperplasia		
BIP	Bronchiolitis obliterans interstitial pneumonitis	ER	Endoplasmic reticulum
		FA	Fatty acid or fluorescent antibody
BM	Bone marrow or basement membrane	FSH	Follicle-stimulating hormone
BMR	Basal metabolic rate		
BPH	Benign prostatic hypertrophy	GC	Gonococcus
		GI	Gastrointestinal
BUN	Blood urea nitrogen	GIT	Gastrointestinal tract
C-19	Number of carbon atoms in the compound (usually in a steroid)	G_O	Cells incapable of undergoing mitosis
		GU	Genitourinary
		GUT	Genitourinary tract
Ca	Calcium or cancer	HAA	Hepatitis-associated antigen (e.g., Australia antigen)
CHF	Congestive heart failure		
CIP	Classic interstitial pneumonitis		
		H and E	Hematoxylin and eosin stain
CNS	Central nervous system		
COBS	Chronic organic brain syndrome	HCG	Human chorionic gonadotropin
CPC	Chronic passive congestion	HDN	Hemolytic disease of the newborn
CPK	Creatine phosphokinase	HIAA	5-Hydroxy indoleacetic acid
CSF	Cerebrospinal fluid		

1

ABBREVIATION	TERM	ABBREVIATION	TERM
HPF	(per) High power field	PAP (smear)	Papanicolaou smear cytology
Hx	History		
IASD	Intra-atrial septal defect	PAS	Periodic acid Schiff stain
IgG, IgA	Immunoglobulin G (for gamma); A (for alpha)	PBI	Protein-bound iodine
IgM	Immunoglobulin M (for mu)	pH	Negative log of hydrogen ion concentration
IH	Infectious hepatitis		
IM	Intramuscular	PID	Pelvic inflammatory disease
IVP	Intravenous pyelogram		
IVSD	Intraventricular-septal defect	PMN	Polymorphonuclear leukocyte, poly, neutrophil
JG	Juxtaglomerular (apparatus or cell)	PNS	Peripheral nervous system
KOH	Potassium hydroxide		
KP	Keratitic precipitates	PPLO	Pleuropneumonia-like organisms
LATS	Long-acting thyroid stimulator	PTH	Parathyroid hormone
LCM	Lymphocytic choriomeningitis	PTAH	Phosphotungstic acid-hematoxylin— stain
LFT	Liver Function Tests		
LH	Luteinizing hormone	Px	Prognosis
LIP	Lymphocyte interstitial pneumonitis	RA	Right atrium or rheumatoid arthritis
LON	League of Nations	RBC	Red blood cell
LV	Left ventricle	RER	Rough endoplasmic reticulum
LVH	Left ventricular hypertrophy	RE (system)	Reticuloendothelial system
MACG	Multiple adenomatous colloid goiter	RHD	Rheumatic heart disease
MAO	Monamine oxidase	RhoGAM	Trade name for anti-Rho(D) antibody used to prevent erythroblastosis fetalis
MEA	Multiple endocrine adenopathies; multiple endocrine adenomas		
MI	Myocardial infarct		
MR	Mental retardation	RNA	Ribonucleic acid
MS	Multiple sclerosis	RV	Right ventricle
MSH	Melanocyte-stimulating hormone	RVH	Right ventricular hypertrophy
NEFA	Nonesterified fatty acids	Rx	Therapy or treatment
		SBE	Subacute bacterial endocarditis
OIP	Oxygen-induced interstitial pneumonitis	SER	Smooth endoplasmic reticulum
OH-CS	Hydroxicorticosteroids	SH	Serum hepatitis
P (waves)	P waves of EKG associated with atrial exudation	SMC	Smooth muscle cell
		S-S	Sulfur to sulfur bonds— covalent
PAP	Pulmonary alveolar proteinosis—lung	Sx	Symptoms

ABBREVIATION	TERM	ABBREVIATION	TERM
T and A	Tonsillectomy and adenoidectomy	UIP	Usual interstitial pneumonitis
TB, TBC	Tuberculosis	URI	Upper respiratory infection
THIN	Thrombosis, hemorrhage, infarct, necrosis	UV	Ultraviolet
T_3	Triiodothyronine	VDRL	Venereal Disease Research Laboratories (test for syphilis)
T_4	Thyroxin		
TSH	Thyroid-stimulating hormone	VMA	Vanillylmandelic acid
TTP	Thrombotic thrombocytogenic purpura	WBC	White blood cell
		WEE	Western equine encephalitis
UCG	Urinary chorionic gonadotropin (test for pregnancy)	X zone	(Androgenic) inner zone of fetal and newborn adrenal gland

1 Skin–Nontumors

DERMATOLOGICAL ALPHABET

Gross

Bulla: An elevated, fluid-containing lesion of the skin *over* 0.5 cm. in diameter
Burrow: A characteristic sign of an animal parasite such as *Sarcoptes scabiei*
Comedo or "blackhead": A plug of secretion retained in a follicle because of closure of its opening by excess cornification
Lichenification: Thickening and exaggeration of *normal* skin markings and of furrows (e.g., neurodermatitis)
Macule: A spot *not* elevated above the skin surface
Nodule: A solid, elevated lesion of the skin *over* 0.5 cm. in diameter
Papule: A solid, elevated lesion of the skin up to 0.5 cm. in diameter
Pustule: An elevated, pus-containing lesion of the skin up to 0.5 cm. in diameter
Vesicle: An elevated, fluid-containing lesion of the skin up to 0.5 cm. in diameter
Wheal: A solid, elevated lesion of the skin formed by transient intense, local, superficial edema

Micro

NOTE: Please review normal skin anatomy in appropriate texts
Acantholysis: Loss of intercellular bridges between epithelial cells with loss of cohesion
Acanthosis: Thickening of prickle layer (stratum spinosum) of skin (often with elongated rete pegs)
Degenerations of skin:
    a. acidophilic = hyaline degeneration, keloids, scars
    b. basophilic = collagen diseases and senile skin
    c. mucoid = skin myxedema
    d. granular = extensive granuloma annulare
Dyskeratosis: Abnormal keratinization of epidermal cells (e.g., with senile keratosis)
Hyperkeratosis: Thickening of the stratum corneum
Papillomatosis: Upward finger-like extensions of dermal papillae and overlying epidermis
Parakeratosis: Maintenance of nuclei in the stratum corneum
Spongiosis: Edema between epithelial cells with increased space between them (elongated intercellular bridges)

UV-INDUCED DNA DAMAGE

Human Diseases Associated With Defective Repair of UV-Caused Damage

	Xeroderma Pigmentosum	*De Sanctis-Cacchione Syndrome*
Heredity	Autosomal recessive	Autosomal recessive
Clinical	1. Exquisite sensitivity to UV light (3000 Å) 2. Gradually deepening skin pigmentation of exposed parts 3. Begins in early childhood	Same skin findings as xeroderma pigmentosum, plus mental retardation, mental defects, dwarfism, and gonadal hypoplasia
Pathology	1. Skin wrinkled, atrophic, shiny 2. Telangiectasia 3. Keratosis and malignancy are common features	
Key Words	1. Basic pathology is lack of UV-activated endonuclease No DNA repair of UV-induced pyrimidine dimers 2. Responds normally to x-ray damage	Etiology same as xeroderma pigmentosum

UV Damage to DNA

Caused by damage to pyrimidine in a single strand of DNA:pyrimidine dimers
1. Cytosine – cytosine
2. Cytosine – thymidine
3. Thymidine – thymidine

Mechanisms of DNA Repair After UV Damage

Type of Repair	Mechanism	White Light Needed	Present In
Photoreactive repair	Monomerization of dimer in situ	Yes	Fish through marsupials
Dark repair	Excision and replication of dimer strand	No	Higher mammals and man

UV Damage (Dimerization)—Mechanism of Repair in Humans

Step	Enzyme	Action
1	UV-activated endonuclease	Causes break in single-strand DNA near a UV-induced dimer
2	Exonuclease	Excision of the single strand of DNA containing the dimer
3	DNA polymerase (repair replication non-Watson-Crick mechanism)	Fills gap with nondimerized pyrimidine
4	DNA ligase	Closes broken strand of DNA

Infections of Skin I

Disease	Etiology	Location	Key Words
Dermatophytosis (general)	Trichophyton, Microsporum and Epidermophyton groups of fungi	Superficial in skin, hair, nails	1. Athlete's foot is the most common type; usually with hyperhidrosis 2. Rate of growth in skin proportional to keratin formation.
Tinea capitis	Most common cause *Microsporum audouni,* also *Microsporum canis*	Scalp	Ringworm
Tinea corporis	Most common cause *Microsporum canis*	Body	Ringworm
Tinea cruris	Most common cause *Epidermophyton floccosum*	Genital area	"Jock itch"
Tinea versicolor (pityriasis versicolor)	Due to *Malassezia furfur*	Usually on trunk, under breasts, etc.	1. Most superficial fungus infection (only in stratum corneum) 2. Culture unnecessary 3. Can only be diagnosed by biopsy or smear; "meatballs in spaghetti" on KOH
Sporotrichosis	Caused by *Sporothrix schenkii*	Hands, arms	1. From rose, barberry and carnations (gardeners) 2. Chancre-like lesion with chain of subcutaneous granulomas which can ulcerate 3. Spores
Candidiasis (thrush, moniliasis)	*Candida albicans*	Mucosal surfaces anywhere, intertriginous areas (perineal, inframammary, axillary)	Opportunistic organism common cause of diaper rash

FUNGAL SKIN DISEASES—GENERAL

1. Id: A hypersensitive reaction to fungi or tuberculosis; *NO* organisms in id lesion
2. Kerion: An abscess due to fungal immunity. Fungi must be found in the lesion, otherwise it is an id or bacterial in etiology. Better prognosis with kerion than id.
3. Wood's light: UV (356 nm.) is helpful for fungal diagnoses because most fungi fluoresce; especially good with tinea capitis and tinea versicolor
4. Special stains: Fungi can be identified by culture and stains on slides (PAS or Gridley). Need to use KOH to dissolve keratin in smears.

Infections of Skin II: Tuberculosis of Skin

Disease	Location	Micro	Key Words
Lupus vulgaris	Maculopapular rash on face	Typical TBC	Apple-jelly nodules (erythema obliterated with slide and pressure) Probe (toothpick) test positive—deep dermal involvement
Erythema induratum	Posterior surface of lower legs	Obliterative vasculitis, perivascular tubercles	History of TBC Almost always in young girls in cold weather Painless, deep lesions, may ulcerate May be related to erythema nodosum

Maculopapulosquamous Diseases

	Psoriasis	*Lichen Planus*	*Pityriasis Rosea*
Etiology	Biochemical abnormality Hereditary—emotional (?)	Infection (?)	Infections Contact (new pajamas)
Clinical	Family history common Pruritus usually slight	Family history common Pruritus severe	Spontaneous cure (8 weeks) No recurrence Lesions follow dermatomes
Incidence	5% of all dermatoses Most common in males, puberty to age 45 Rare in blacks	Less common than psoriasis More common in women Usually after age 30	
Location	Most common on EXTENSOR surfaces, knees, elbows, and scalp, pitting nails common	Most common on FLEXOR surfaces and inner cheek opposite 1st molar, spares face	Abrupt symmetrical eruption on trunk
Pathology			
Gross	Silver scale plaques Point bleeding when removed	VIOLACEOUS, flat-top (often infected), NONSCALY lesion	Erythematous, nonscaly eruption
Micro	Munro's microabscesses–stratum corneum Test tube rete pegs Parakeratosis	Sawtooth rete pegs Platelike acanthosis Many round cells in upper dermis Liquefaction of basal epidermis	Lymphocytes in outer dermis Spongiosis Acanthosis Parakeratosis
Key words	1. Must differentiate from parapsoriasis 2. Koebner's phenomenon (lesions develop in a scratch mark) positive 3. Often associated with arthritis or ulcerative colitis 4. Now being treated with methotrexate and UV light 5. High DNA turnover, cell proliferation	1. No arthritis or ulcerative colitis 2. Koebner's phenomenon positive	1. Herald patch precedes 2. Must do VDRL to rule out syphilis

Chronic Vesiculobullous Disorders

	Pemphigus Vulgaris	Bullous Pemphigoid	Dermatitis Herpetiformis
Etiology	? Autoimmune, IgG in intercellular space	? Autoimmune, IgG along epithelial BM	Atopic dermatitis or infantile eczema plus herpes simplex
Clinical			
Age	50+	Elderly adults	Usually adults
Location	Abdomen, scalp, groin, mouth	Generalized, with or without oral lesions	Scapulas, trunk, sacrum
Lesions	Normal skin at edge of bullae	Erythema at edge usually	Erythema at base of lesion
Weight loss	4+	+−	None
Pruritus	0	+−	4+
Oral pain	4+	None	None
Grouping	No	No	Yes
Pathology	1. Acantholysis with intraepidermal, suprabasal bullae 2. Have basal layer below bullae 3. Heals without scar	1. No acantholysis 2. Subepithelial bullae 3. *NO* basal layer below bullae	1. Subepidermal bullae 2. *NO* basal layer below bullae 3. Mononuclears and eosinophils abundant
Key Words	1. Fatal if not treated 2. Nikolsky's sign (denuded area or blister with skin twist) positive 3. May develop into exfoliative dermatitis 4. Plasma protein often LOW 5. Anti-intracellular substance on FA of skin biopsy	1. *NOT* fatal by itself 2. Must be distinguished from erythema multiforme, bullosum, and others 3. Spontaneous remission frequent 4. May be associated with internal malignancy, especially of ovary 5. Anti-BM by FA in skin biopsy	1. In pregnancy it is called herpes gestationalis 2. Often sulfonamide-responsive.

Eczematous Dermatoses

Contact Dermatitis	Infantile Eczema	Stasis Dermatitis	Exfoliative Dermatitis
Etiology			
External contact, in sensitive patients, to 1. Allergen 2. Light 3. Primary irritants	Temporary allergy to environmental factors	Vascular insufficiency Arteriolar obstruction and varicosities	Most common secondary to psoriasis May be spontaneous, also with heavy-metal treatment
Clinical			
Edema, vesicle, pustule, crust	Erythema, edema, vesicles, scaling, pruritus, lichenification	Eczematous, pigmented rash, lower leg, may ulcerate later	Gradually spreading universal erythema (red Indian) Hot, dry skin with fever, pruritus, scaling Enlarged lymph nodes
Incidence			
Usually in younger age group	In infants to age 2	Usually in older age group	Any age group
Location			
Lesions usually focal in areas of contact	Usually on face or flexor surfaces	Most common above medial malleolus	Generalized

(Continued on facing page)

Eczematous Dermatoses *(continued)*

Contact Dermatitis	*Infantile Eczema*	*Stasis Dermatitis*	*Exfoliative Dermatitis*

Pathology

Acute: vesicles, spongiosis, edema, vasodilation, neutrophils *Subacute:* acanthosis, hyperkeratosis and eosinophils *Chronic:* hyperkeratosis, parakeratosis, mononuclear cells	Nonspecific dermatitis; same as contact dermatitis	Edema, hyperkeratosis and chronic inflammation Hemosiderin in skin Increased melanin pigment	Nonspecific dermatitis, hyperkeratosis, acanthosis If caused by psoriasis or lymphoma, can see them

Key Words

1. Cured when irritant is removed 2. Patch test to diagnose	1. If present over age 2 is atopic dermatitis 2. May develop asthma as adults 3. *NO* smallpox vaccination, may get generalized vaccinia 4. With herpes simplex may get eczema herpeticum	Common in people who stand a lot (policemen, salesmen)	1. Signifies a lymphoma or leukemia in 25% of cases 2. Outcome frequently fatal 3. Sezary syndrome

Urticaria, Toxic Erythemas, and Drug Eruptions

Urticaria (Hives)	Erythema Multiforme	Erythema Nodosum	Dermatitis Medicamentosa

Etiology

Allergy to food, drugs or other agents Excess histamine	Allergy (?), drugs (?), herpes simplex (Hebra)	Hypersensitivity to streptococci, pneumococci, coccidiomycosis, drugs	Due to hypersensitivity, any drug

Clinical

1. *Circumscribed* area of edema, wheals, often surrounded by erythema 2. Most common on trunk 3. Dermatographism is common	Three types: 1. *Idiopathic (Hebra):* herpes simplex (?) —circular red lesion often with "iris" or "target"— face, back, hands, lips 2. *Symptomatic:* erythematous, edematous, circular lesions mostly on trunk; erythema marginatum of rheumatic fever is a type 3. *Stevens-Johnson:* high fever, prostration, involvement of conjunctiva and oral mucosa; usually on genitals, hands and feet; may cause blindness and death	1. Symmetrical, nodular, erythematous, painful swelling on extensor aspect of legs 2. NO ulcerations 3. Low-grade fever common	1. Most commonly maculopapular rash with few bullae; barbiturates most common cause 2. Penicillin usually urticarial 3. Anaphylaxis may develop

Pathology

1. Perivesicular edema, flattened rete pegs and spongiosis 2. Few perivascular lymphocytes	Bullae, vesicles, papules, macules; acute, subacute and chronic dermatitis	Vasculitis involving fat with epithelioid cells, giant cells, and, later, foam cells	Nonspecific inflammation, occasionally with rash

Key Words

Hereditary angioedema, formerly	Nonspecific perivascular inflammatory cells	May be related to Weber-Christian disease, relapsing	1. Rash disappears when drug is stopped

(Continued on facing page)

Urticaria, Toxic Erythemas, and Drug Eruptions *(continued)*

Urticaria (Hives)	Erythema Multiforme	Erythema Nodosum	Dermatitis Medicamentosa
angioneurotic edema, is a variant, —due to absence of Cls, Inh. (complement inhibitor deficiency), an autosomal dominant hereditary disease which may have laryngeal edema as a cause of death	May involve mucosal surfaces	nonsuppurative panniculitis	2. Fixed drug reactions in same place with same drug; phenolphthalein most common cause of fixed reaction 3. No lab or skin test available

Acne and the Seborrheic Dermatoses

	Acne Vulgaris	Rosacea	Seborrheic Dermatitis
Definition	"Ugly points"	"Rosy, pale"	"Tallow flow"
Etiology	1. Hormonal imbalance 2. Normal physiology (?)	1. Vasomotor instability in seborrheic patients 2. Menopause (?)	Unknown, (?) endocrine dysfunction, emotional
Clinical	May be severe with scars and pits Most cure spontaneously by age 16	NO comedones Rhinophyma— hypertrophic rosacea	Mildest form-dandruff *Most* common skin lesion Cradle cap in infants
Incidence	Most common skin lesion of adolescents (occurs in 75%)	Most common in women	Common in obese patients
Location	Comedones on face, upper chest and back	Red, flushed middle 1/3 of face in middle age	Most common on scalp, eyebrows, intertriginous areas
Pathology	1. Dilated, plugged, ruptured sebaceous glands 2. Acute folliculitis due to bacteria and picking 3. Chronic granulomatous disease with SCARRING	1. Dilated sebaceous glands with chronic inflammation 2. Rhinophyma— hypertrophy of glands and connective tissue	1. Sebaceous glands unremarkable 2. Nonspecific inflammation characterized by: spongiosis, hyperkeratosis, parakeratosis, few round cells
Key words	1. Rx: high-dose vitamin A 2. NO malignancy unless treated with radiation 3. Now often Rxed with antibiotics 4. C. acnes may be etiology	1. Hypochlorhydria is common 2. Rhinophyma more common in alcoholic men	1. Acne, rosacea, and psoriasis may be complications 2. May have alopecia and pityriasis capitis or dry scalp

2 Skin Tumors

GENERAL

1. Arise from germinal epithelial or basal cells
2. Most probably represent hamartomas
3. Almost all are BENIGN
4. All rarely undergo malignant degeneration
5. If malignant, rarely metastasize widely

Morphology of Benign Adnexal Skin Tumors

Classification	Organic	Organoid	Suborganoid	Nonorganoid
	(Organic hamartoma)	(Partial organ hamartoma)	(Benign epithelioma)	(Basal cell carcinoma)
Some examples With hair	1. Pigmentary, hairy nevus	1. Folliculoma	1. Calcifying epithelioma of Malherbe	1. Keratotic
Sebaceous	2. Sebaceous nevus	2. Sebaceous adenoma	2. Eccrine poroma	2. Cystic
Apocrine	3. Apocrine nevus	3. Syringocyst- adenoma	3. Trichoepi- thelioma	3. Adenoid

All may differentiate to: (a) hair, (b) sebaceous structures, (c) apocrine structures, (d) eccrine structures, (e) sheets of basal cells

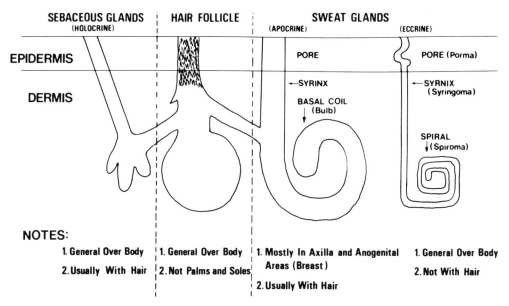

Fig. 2–1. Tumor origins in the skin.

Common Benign Cystic Tumors of Skin

	Sebaceous Cyst	Epidermal Inclusion Cyst
Etiology	Plugged duct, congenital	Congenital, surgical, infectious or traumatic
Clinical	Commonly mistaken for epidermal inclusion cyst	Most common cyst of skin
Location	Almost exclusively on scalp	Usually on head or back. Pilonidal cyst is special type (males 10:1), occurs over sacrum
Pathology	Cyst lined with sebaceous cells, filled with sebum, bad odor	Cyst lined with squamous epithelium. Contains keratin
Key words	Both surrounded by inflammatory cells with foreign body reaction due to rupture or picking; both may have common origin and do not become malignant	

Common Nevi

Type	Pathology	Special Key Features
Intradermal	Nests of nevus cells in dermis NO junctional component	Does NOT become malignant Occurs at any age MOST common nevus
Junctional	Nests of nevus cells *AT* dermoepidermal junction	Malignant potential but malignancy uncommon
Compound	Intradermal nests of cells with junctional activity	Malignant potential but rarely malignant
Juvenile (spindle cell)	Compound nevi with spindle cells, giant (muscle) cells, some separation of cells	Most common on face in prepubertal age group Looks malignant, behaves benignly Juvenile melanoma
Blue	Blue color on gross Location: deep dermis Nevus cell nests	Looks and is benign Also called Jadassohn-Tieche nevus Usually in children on extremities
Mongolian spot	Spindle-shaped, dopa-positive cells in mid-dermis	Sacral region, present at birth Most common in Asiatics Probably a variety of blue nevus

Common Primary Malignant Tumors of Skin

	Squamous Cell Carcinoma	Basal Cell Carcinoma Rodent Ulcer	Malignant Melanoma
Etiology	Common sequela of burns, sunlight, UV, x-ray May begin as senile keratosis or Bowen's disease, corps ronds	Sunlight, x-ray Hamartoma	Arises from junctional nevus (?)
Most common locations	Exposed areas, lower face, backs, hands	Face above corner of mouth, ears	Lower extremities, foot, head Melanotic whitlow in nails
Gross	Small, ulcerated, firm NO pigment	Ulcerated, often pigmented	Usually pigmented May be amelanotic Satellite nodules
Micro	Squamous cells with or without pearls	Nests of cells—peripheral "picket fence"	Anaplastic nevus cells Loss of cohesiveness Invasion
Special features	1. Metastasis not common	1. NO metastasis 2. Commonly recur	1. Metastasis early and far

(Continued on facing page)

Common Primary Malignant Tumors of Skin *(continued)*

	Squamous Cell Carcinoma	Basal Cell Carcinoma Rodent Ulcer	Malignant Melanoma
	2. Basal cell and squamous carcinoma together are most common tumors overall in humans; rarely cause death 3. 5% with Bowen's disease have internal malignancies	3. Often multicentric in origin	2. May be dormant for years 3. Hutchinson's melanotic freckle (lentigo maligna) premalignant 1/3 become invasive 4. Superficial melanoma has better prognosis than deep; overall 25% 5-year survival 5. The "syphilis" of tumors

Less Common Primary Malignant Tumors of Skin

	Kaposi's Sarcoma	Mycosis Fungoides
Most common locations	Begins on foot, especially on great toe (U.S.A.)	Primary in skin
Clinical	Common in Africa, rare in U.S.A. Purplish-blue lesions, may become generalized	Malignant lymphoreticular disease Pruritic, ulcerated, nodular with diffuse erythema Usually occurs in middle age
Pathology	Basically a vascular sarcoma, proliferated, malignant fibroblasts and blood vessels Patients have a high incidence of lymphomas	Pleomorphic reticulum-like cells reminiscent of Hodgkin's disease, with microabscesses (Pautrier's), polys, eosinophils, lymphocytes, histiocytes, giant cells and pseudogiant cells Not the same as lymphoma or leukemia cutis (these have distinctive histology)

Seborrheic Keratosis vs. Senile Keratosis

	Seborrheic Keratosis (Basal Cell Papilloma)	Senile Keratosis
Location	Most common on trunk	On exposed areas: face, backs of hands
Malignant potential	NO (0)	Yes; premalignant (squamous cell carcinoma Grade ½) Also seen with arsenic exposure
Pathology	Basal cell papilloma, cysts with keratin surrounded by epidermis, hyperkeratosis with acanthosis	Dyskeratosis, hyperkeratosis, mitotic activity, basophilic degeneration of collagen
Key words	Superficial, greasy, pigmented, "stuck-on" lesions, often multiple	Not superficial, pigmented. Usually singular

Viral Tumors of the Skin

	Verruca	Molluscum Contagiosum
Clinical	Three types: 1. Vulgaris (? Papovavirus) 2. Plantaris (plantar wart) 3. Plana—flat (juvenile wart) Fluorescence with Wood's light	NO fluorescence with Wood's light Poxvirus, waxy-white, globular, usually under 1 cm. in size
Location	*Verruca vulgaris:* (commonest) usually hands ("toads") *Plantar wart:* on sole of foot—painful Flat wart: on hands and faces of children	Most common on trunk and eyelids of children and athletes
Pathology	Vulgaris: localized papillomatosis, hyperkeratosis, parakeratosis, intra-nuclear eosinophilic inclusions; vacuolated balloon cells in granular layer Plantaris: same histology as in vulgaris but more hyperkeratosis Plana: similar to vulgaris but less keratin and acanthosis	Molluscum bodies, eosinophilic, in cytoplasm of epithelial cells, also acanthosis, parakeratosis, and some hyperkeratosis
Key words	Does not become malignant	Heals spontaneously Does not become malignant

XANTHOMATOUS LESIONS OF THE SKIN

General

1. All characterized by focal or diffuse nodular deposits
2. Associated with familial hyperlipidemias, and lipidemias
3. Secondary to arteriosclerosis, biliary cirrhosis and nephrosis

Micro

Foam cells, Touton giant cells, histiocytes

Special Types of Xanthomatous Lesions of the Skin

	Xanthelasma	Xanthoma Tuberosum	Xanthoma Diabeticorum
Location	Eyelids	Joints, palms, soles and along tendon sheaths, extensor surfaces	Usually on flexor surfaces
Description	Yellow plaques associated with hypercholesterolemia	Yellowish nodules	Small, papular lesions
Key words	Also called xanthelasma palpebrarum	Seen with either primary or secondary hyperlipidemia	Associated with diabetes under poor control

3 Pulmonary Review, Bronchitis and Pneumonia

THE LUNGS

BLOOD VESSELS OF THE LUNG

Arteries (2 Sets)

1. Bronchial: multiple along bronchi
2. Pulmonary: act as end arteries
3. Arteriole: smooth muscle controls blood flow
4. Capillary: 1:1 ratio of air to blood spaces (capillary dance)

Veins

Single set of veins (pulmonary), NO bronchial veins in lung lobule

Lymphatics (3 sets)

1. Peribronchial: periarterial lymphatics
2. Interstitial system of lymphatics, drain lobules, follow pulmonary veins
3. Pleural lymphatic system, drain from pleura

CARTILAGE OF THE LUNG

Normal

Hyaline cartilage present in decreasing amounts from the larynx to the bronchi that are greater than 1 mm. in diameter; hardens after birth

Pathological Changes

Chondromalacia, lobar emphysema in infants
Ossification, old age
Chondritis, tuberculosis
Ochronosis, stained black (homogentisic acid)

PATHOLOGIC CAVITIES IN THE LUNG

Abscess

1. Rough walls
2. Connect with MANY bronchi
3. TBC cavities connect with MANY bronchi
4. MOST common location of abscess cavities = right upper lobe, posterior segment

Bullae

1. Smooth walls
2. Connect with ONE bronchus
3. Giant bullae—surgical emphysema

GLANDS OF THE LUNG

Normal

Mucous glands are normal, decreasing in amount down bronchial tree

Pathological Changes

1. Hyperplasia + hypertrophy: asthma and chronic bronchitis
2. Metaplasia: anaplasia, tumors
3. Biochemical abnormalities: mucoviscidosis—asthma

MUSCLE OF THE LUNG

Normal

Smooth muscle is wound spirally around bronchioles, blood vessels, and lymphatics

Pathological Changes

Muscle usually increased with diseases that cause increased tension on lung
1. Hyperplasia + hypertrophy
   a. asthma
   b. bronchiectasis early; late, atrophy with chronic bronchitis
   c. leiomyomatosis, muscular cirrhosis
   d. honeycombing, enlarged distal air spaces with excess interstitial thickening
2. Atrophy, SCAR, bronchiectasis late

NERVES OF THE LUNG

1. Scarce, and hard to find in lung parenchyma without special techniques
2. People over 40 often get tiny carotid-body-like tumors
3. Nerves that look like taste buds often seen
4. Some nerves around bronchi and along pleura

ALVEOLAR STRUCTURE

ALVEOLAR AIR BARRIER

500 million alveoli per lung; alveolar volume: capillary volume = 1:1

ALVEOLAR CELL TYPES

1. Type I, membranous: pneumocytes, most numerous, lining cell of alveoli
2. Type II, granular: pneumocytes, electron-dense lamellar bodies which contain surfactant (reduces surface tension), a phospholipoprotein (dipalmityl-lecithin)
3. Type III, phagocytic: pneumocytes (modified macrophages), can burrow through alveolar wall, have many lysosomes and cytosomes

Comparison of Alveolar Cell Types

Property	Membranous Pneumocyte (Type I)	Granular Pneumocyte (Type II)	Phagocytic Pneumocyte (Type III)
Phagocytosis	+ −	+ −	4
Inclusions	+ −	+ −	4+
Lamellar bodies	+ −	4+	+ −
Ferritin (hemosiderin)	+ −	+ −	4+

BRONCHIAL EPITHELIAL CELL TYPES

1. Mucin-producing (goblet) cells: excess mucin leads to obstruction
2. Ciliated cells: cilia beat toward mouth with coordinated beat; rate of propulsion-several cm./min. Inhibited by: SO_2 (1.6 p.p.m.), cigarette smoke
3. Intermediate cells or primitive basal cells; multipotential
4. Myoepithelial cells: close to basement membrane, present in very small numbers
5. Secretory cells with granules; same as Kulchitsky cells in GIT (serotonin), source of carcinoid type of adenoma
6. Brush cell; contains lots of glycogen, mostly in terminal bronchioles; "sugar tumor"

Etiologic Factors in Bronchiectasis

Factor Associated	Number of Cases
Pneumonitis	66
Pertussis	10
Other infections	8
Foreign body	6
T and A (tonsillectomy and adenoidectomy)	5
Kartagener's syndrome	3
Silicosis	1
Cases with KNOWN factors	99
Cases with UNKNOWN factors	114
TOTAL cases	213
Percent with known associated factors	49%

Summary: The etiology of about 50% of bronchiectasis cases UNKNOWN

Bronchiectasis and Chronic Bronchitis

Parameter	Bronchiectasis	Chronic Bronchitis
Etiology	UNKNOWN Chronic inflammation, congenital (?)	Chemical and bacterial irritants, sulfur dioxide, cigarette smoking, congenital (?)
Pathogenesis	Associated with whooping cough, fibrocystic disease of pancreas, and chronic sinusitis	Excess mucus secretion, inhibited cilia, allergy
Clinical		History of smoking common
Incidence	Common in children and young adults 50% have onset before age 20 No sex predilection	Most common in older adults, rare in children More common in males and in England
Symptoms	Cough up large amounts of foul-smelling sputum, especially in A.M.	Cough with abundant sputum, dyspnea, "blue bloater" terminally
Pathology		
Location	3rd and 4th order bronchi, usually in lower lobes, left greater than right	Proximal bronchi most severely affected, also bronchioles
Gross	Dilation of bronchi to pleura Types: (1) saccular, (2) tubular, (3) mixed	Edema, excess mucus with small lumen of bronchi
Micro	Cysts and chronic inflammation, scarring around bronchi	Excess mucus with increased thickness of bronchial glands and loss of cilia Reid index increased = *mucous gland thickness*/total thickness of bronchial wall (normal up to 0.35)
Special features	1. Kartagener's syndrome: sinusitis, situs inversus, bronchiectasis 2. Clubbing of fingers	1. With fibrous proliferation get bronchiolitis obliterans 2. May be associated with emphysema 3. Squamous metaplasia and carcinoma may occur 4. Cor pulmonale is common sequela

Alveolar Pneumonias

	Bronchopneumonia	Lobar Pneumonia
Etiology	Bacteria: strep, staph, gram-negatives	Bacteria: pneumococcus (*Streptococcus pneumoniae*)
Incidence	Most common in old and young	Common in middle age
Gross	Focal	Classic hepatizations, entire lobe involved
Micro	Polys in alveoli with necrosis	Polys in alveoli, necrosis rare, necrosis with Type 3 and 8 penumococcus
Complications	Abscess, empyema Organization - scar	Abscess Empyema
Special feature	Vasculitis when due to Pseudomonas	Usually does not organize

Special Pneumonias

Lipoid Pneumonia	Pneumocystis	Pulmonary Alveolar Proteinosis (PAP)	Cytomegalic Inclusion-Interstitial Pneumonia
Endogenous: Common with bronchogenic carcinoma, golden brown color, lipid-laden (cholesterol) macrophages *Exogenous:* Nose drops, inhalation etc., unsaturated, short-chain, and free, fatty acids are most irritating	*Pneumocystis carinii*, protozoan is cause Most common in children and debilitated adults Find organism in lungs with Grocott stain May be confused with PAP Foamy material with few inflammatory cells	Amorphous material in alveoli Abnormal (?) surfactant No significant inflammatory cell infiltrate Negative Grocott stain Probably NOT a pneumonia but a pneumoconiosis	Cytomegalic inclusion virus Common in infants and debilitated persons, especially with immunosuppressive therapy and in immunologic cripples Micro: large pneumocytes with large intranuclear inclusions

Interstitial Pneumonias

Usual or Classical (UIP or CIP)	Bronchiolitis Obliterans (BIP)	Oxygen-Induced (OIP)	Desquamative (DIP)
Etiology			
Viruses, PPLO Chemicals: Hg Radiation Diseases: uremia, rheumatic fever	Nitrogen dioxide; silo-filler's disease	Iatrogenic (excess oxygen therapy)	UNKNOWN (silica, graphite, talc inhalation?)
Incidence			
Any age	Rare	Uncommon	Rare
Gross			
Firm, slimy, meaty lungs	Firm, slimy, meaty lungs	Firm, slimy, meaty, lungs	Firm, slimy, meaty lungs
Micro			
Classic: diffuse necrosis of alveolar epithelium, mononuclear cells in thickened septa with rare polys and edema in alveoli, hyaline membranes may occur *Late:* interstitial proliferation, honey-combing	Same as UIP, but with marked bronchiolar alveolar proliferation and obstruction	Same as UIP except that hyaline membrane tends to be more common and more pronounced	Interstitial inflammation with alveoli filled with Type II pneumocytes Honeycombing less frequent than in UIP
Complications			
Bacterial pneumonia often superimposed	Bacterial pneumonia often superimposed	Bacterial pneumonia often superimposed	Bacterial pneumonia often superimposed
Special Features			
1. Often leads to honeycombing 2. Alveolar capillary block occurs; key symptom = tachypnea 3. Symptoms worse than x-ray shows	History of working around newly filled silo	History of 1–2 days' oxygen therapy, especially with a closed system	1. Steroids treat it 2. Other variants: LIP (lymphocyte); GIP (giant cell), PIP (plasma cell); not treated with steroids

4 Tumors and Pneumoconioses

Common Lesions of the Larynx

Polyp	Papilloma	Carcinoma
Clinical		
1. Most common in smokers and those who use their voices often 2. Singer's nodule 3. Sx: progressive hoarseness	1. Hoarseness 2. Airway obstruction	1. Usually in adults over 40; male : female ratio = 10:1 2. Sx: hoarseness, respiratory obstruction, hemoptysis
Gross		
1. Smooth, rounded, pedunculated; rarely more than 1 cm. in diameter 2. Usually on true cord 3. May be ulcerated	1. Succulent, friable, raspberry-like; rarely more than 1 cm. in diameter 2. Usually on true cord	1. Small plaque-like lesions 2. Usually on true vocal cords INTRINSIC 3. May occur in piriform sinus or false cord, EXTRINSIC
Micro		
1. Early: loose connective-myxomatous tissue core with maturation to collagenized SCAR 2. Late: hyalinized SCAR	1. Finger-like projections 2. Hyperkeratosis 3. Atypical epithelial proliferation 4. Premalignant	1. 95% are squamous cell carcinomas 2. Others adenocarcinomas
Special Features		
Does not predispose to malignancy	1. Multiple papillomas in prepubertal children often regress, rarely become malignant 2. Single, in adults, often becomes malignant	1. Intrinsic better prognosis than extrinsic 2. 25%–35% overall 5-year survival rate

Less Common Lesions of the Nasopharynx

	Nasopharyngeal Fibroma (Juvenile Fibroma)	Lymphoepithelioma (Schmincke's Tumor)
Clinical	Most common in pubertal males	Most common in nasopharynx, primary often not discovered, most common in young males
Pathological	Dense fibrous tissue with many blood vessels	Composed of malignant squamous cells and lymphoid elements
Key words	1. Often regress spontaneously 2. Bleeds profusely with surgery 3. Rarely if ever metastasizes 4. Tends to behave as a malignant tumor in adults	1. Usually first diagnosed by metastases in nodes 2. Common in Chinese in Formosa 3. Most commonly arises in the fossa of Rosenmuller

LUNG CANCER

Occurrence

1. More common in males than females; female incidence rising
2. Most common carcinoma causing death in males in U.S.A.
3. Peak age incidence = 60 yrs.

Etiology

1. 10 to 20 times more common in cigarette smokers than in nonsmokers
2. Occupational: a definite etiological occurrence seen between lung cancer and occupational exposure to arsenic, uranium (miners), nickel and chromate fumes, and asbestos (20% of patients with asbestosis die of bronchogenic carcinoma)
3. Environmental: higher incidence in areas with air pollution (e.g., 3,4-benzpyrene, 3,12-benzpyrene, coal tar fumes, radioactive substances)

Site of Origin

1. Right lung	52%	
Left lung	48%	
2. Central 1st and 2nd order bronchi	50%	
3. Bronchi beyond 2nd order	30% (bronchogenic)	
4. Peripheral scar in alveolar cell carcinoma	20%	

Spread of Metastasis

1. Most common site of spread is tracheobronchial nodes   70%
2. Patients who die of lung cancer without its spreading outside the thoracic cavity   30%
3. Most common sites of metastasis are: brain   20%
                                            bone   20%
                                            adrenals   50%

Signs and Symptoms

Key word: LATE
Cough: 75%
Weight loss: 40%
Chest pain: 35%
Dyspnea: 20%

Tumors and Tumorlike Conditions of the Lung I

Squamous Cell Carcinoma	Undifferentiated Carcinoma	Adenocarcinoma	Alveolar Cell Carcinoma
Etiology			
Cigarette smoking, air pollution	Cigarette smoking, air pollution	Unknown, usually peripheral, common in scars "scar carcinoma"; also in mucous glands	Unknown, peripheral, multifocal, often occurs in area with previous honeycombing
Gross			
White, firm mass in 1st and 2nd order bronchi		White mass, usually peripheral	Diffuse, mucoid, grayish-white columnar cells
Micro			
Squamous cells in sheets with pearls	Several patterns (e.g., oat cells, giant cells) No pearls or glands	Malignant glands and stroma	Alveoli with late destruction of alveolar walls
Key Words			
Most common bronchogenic	2nd most common	3rd most common	Least common lung cancer
Incidence			
More common in males than females		Females equal to males	
Prognosis			
10% 5-year survival	Poorest prognosis 3% 5-year survival	Best prognosis, distinct metastasis, less common than with other bronchogenic carcinomas 12% 5-year survival	Multicentric origin makes removal difficult
Overall 5-year survival of all lung cancers is 8%			Must distinguish from metastatic adenocarcinoma Resembles jagziekte, a viral disease (a tumor of Type II pneumocytes in sheep)

Tumors and Tumorlike Conditions of the Lungs II (Bronchial Adenomas)

	Carcinoid	Cylindromatous (Adenoid Cystic Type)
Etiology	Unknown	Unknown
Histogenesis	Kulchitsky cell	Mucous gland reserve cell
Occurrence	90% of all bronchial adenomas	10% of all bronchial adenomas
Symptoms	Bronchial obstruction, cough and infection in both	
	Flushing, blushing, cyanosis, diarrhea due to excess serotonin May occur without liver metastasis because MAO is in lung	
Gross	White, firm nodule in bronchus	
Micro	Nest of argentaffin cells	Sheets and cords—cysts, glands
Key words	1. Diagnose with 5-HIAA in urine 2. Always some tumor left below epithelium 3. Heart lesions on right side of heart; Early: pure mast cells Later: fibrosis of tricuspid valve 4. Rarely metastasizes	1. Adenoid cystic pattern, identical with adenoid cystic tumors elsewhere (e.g., salivary glands and oral cavity) 2. Tends to be more proximal, more malignant, more iceberg-like, than carcinoid 3. Infrequently metastasizes

Tumors and Tumorlike Conditions of the Lungs III (Mesotheliomas)

Type I	Type II	Type III
1. Benign 2. Focal, nodular 3. Thought to be fibromas (?) 4. NO relation to asbestosis 5. Resection cures	1. Malignant 2. Most common 3. Diffuse, mixed sarcoma and mesothelial cells 4. Common in asbestosis, may see asbestos bodies 5. Mesothelioma of peritoneum tends to have more glands than pleural lesions	1. Focally INVASIVE 2. Rarest type 3. May recur after resection 4. Intermediate tumor (?)

SPECIAL TOPICS: LUNGS

Benign Tumor

Hamartoma: MOST common benign tumor of lung
Fibroma: very rare
Chemodectoma: "Zellballen" carotid-body-like tumors, rare, tiny, adults ONLY
Sclerosing hemangioma: uncommon
Benign clear cell tumor (9 cases): "sugar" tumor; much glycogen in cells, arises from 6th cell type or brush cells in bronchi
Teratoma: *never* seen as primary in lung

Coin Lesions

Single lesion on x-ray, round, size of quarter to half-dollar
1/3 granulomas, usually TBC
1/3 hamartomas
1/3 other tumors, usually malignant

Hormonal and Other Physiologic Effects of Pulmonary Tumors

1. *Most common* is inappropriate ACTH-like secretion (17-OH-CS); not inhibited by dexamethasone—in about 10% of lung carcinomas, especially common with tracheal involvement, most common with oat cell pattern
2. Inappropriate ADH secretion (decreased plasma osmolality and increased urine osmolality), most common with oat cell pattern
3. Excess parathormone (PTH) commonly associated with lung tumors, PTH also associated with breast and kidney tumors
4. Carcinoid syndrome may be seen with malignant lung tumors, with oat cell tumors as well as with carcinoid adenoma
5. Acanthosis nigricans, dermatomyositis
6. Neuromyopathic syndromes: muscular atrophy, loss of Purkinje cells and granular cells in cerebellum
7. 2% of lung cancers show peripheral neuritis
8. Reagan: heat-stable alkaline phosphatase in 4% of malignant tumors

GRANULOMATOUS PNEUMOCONIOSES

Silicosis

1. Particles
   1–3 microns
2. High incidence of TBC associated
3. Mechanism: degradation of lysosomal and cell membranes by hydrogen bonding
4. Smaller lesions, more peripheral than asbestosis
5. No increase in carcinoma of lung

Asbestosis

1. Asbestos = mineral with fibrous cleavage
   Chrysolite = white asbestos
   Tremolite = talc, more refined
2. Blue velvet pneumonitis, amphetamine and talc, talc emboli
3. High incidence of associated bronchogenic carcinoma and mesotheliomas
4. Asbestos bodies = asbestos covered with iron, stains iron, NOT asbestos itself
5. Frequently found in residential air ducts

Berylliosis

1. Interstitial pneumonitis
2. Double-laminated bodies = *conchoidal bodies*
3. Granulomatous disease, nonhealing
4. Previously from fluorescent lights; now primarily from industrial exposure

Drugs and Others

1. *Hexamethonium* = interstitial fibrosis and hyaline membranes
2. *Maple bark stripper's disease—Cryptostroma corticale*
   Fungus occurs in lumber mills
3. *Bagassosis*—stalk dust, in sugar cutters
4. *Byssinosis*—cotton dust
5. *Fiberglass pneumonitis,* diffuse multilayered alveolar lining, fiberglass in clear spaces
6. *Farmer's lung fungus (Aspergillus fumigatus* and others) moldy hay-sarcoid-like lesion
7. For additional information, see Hypersensitivity Pneumonitis in Sisson, J.A.: Handbook of Clinical Pathology. p. 487.

MISCELLANEOUS PULMONARY DISEASES OF UNKNOWN ETIOLOGIES

Eosinophilic Granuloma

1. 200 cases at AFIP
2. Focal interstitial granulomas
3. Essential cell = histiocyte in interstitium with few eosinophils
4. Pneumothorax very common
5. May regress spontaneously
6. 5%–10% have extrapulmonary disease
7. Steroids may treat

Essential Pulmonary Hemosiderosis

1. Most common in children
2. Fibrosis, hemosiderin-laden macrophages
3. Hemosiderin NOT available to bone marrow, often have hypochromic, microcytic anemia
4. May mistake for DIP, iron stain differentiates
5. Cannot be distinguished from secondary hemosiderosis
6. Goodpasture's syndrome = pulmonary hemorrhage with acute (usually proliferative, AGBM antibody) glomerulonephritis

Loffler's Syndrome

1. Transient eosinophilia
2. Granulomas with central fibrinoid necrosis in lungs with lipid-laden macrophages
3. Some eosinophils may be in lesion
4. Necrotizing vasculitis
5. Probably a variant of eosinophilic granuloma

Hamman-Rich Syndrome

1. Rapidly progressive, diffuse, pulmonary fibrosis
2. Probably a variant of UIP
3. Term little used now

Wegener's Granulomatosis

1. Necrotizing granulomatous arteritis of lungs, upper respiratory tract, and kidney
2. Probably a variant of polyarteritis nodosa

5 Emphysema

COR PULMONALE

Definition

Right ventricular hypertrophy resulting from disease of the structure or function of the lungs, except when due to left ventricular hypertrophy or congenital heart disease.

Anatomic Criteria

1. Right ventricular wall over 5 mm. thickness
2. Right ventricular weight over 65 g. when dissected away from left heart

EMPHYSEMA

Definition

Distal air spaces more than 1 mm. in diameter (Greek—to puff up)

Historic Classifications

Vesicular, bullous, senile

Normal Distal Air Space Diameters

Child: 0.3 mm.
Middle age: 0.5 mm.
Old age: 0.7 mm.

Etiology

Key factor is air trapping with dilatation of distal air spaces

Some Factors Causing Air Trapping

1. *Traction* (pull from without) usually compensatory to:
    a. atelectasis
    b. fibrosis
    c. surgical ablation of lung tissue
2. *Obstruction of air passages* (push from within) by:
    a. mucus
    b. muscle spasm
    c. muscle hyperplasia (asthma)
    d. bronchial fibrosis, external intramural (e.g., bronchiolitis obliterans)
    e. valving, Ball valve phenomenon
3. *Destruction*
    Necrosis, atrophy and enzymes (e.g., trypsin—antitrypsin)

32

4. *Loss of elasticity* (e.g., old garter) elastase-inhibitor deficiency
   a. 1/3 of recoil due to elastic tissue
   b. 2/3 of recoil due to surface tension

Some Other Factors Associated With the Etiology of Emphysema

Increased incidence of emphysema is associated with:
1. *Industrial exposure:* hematite dust, coal dust (miner's lung, black lung disease)
2. *Previous infection: Hemophilus influenzae* pneumonia
3. *Environment:* cigarette smoking (probably an aggravating factor—nitrogen dioxide exposure)
4. *Congenital: lobar emphysema*
   Key words: In children due to softening of cartilage, chondromalacia (looks like fetal cartilage), crowing respirations

ALPHA-1 ANTITRYPSIN DEFICIENCY AND EMPHYSEMA

Principle

1. Deficiency of alpha-1 antitrypsin allows trypsinlike enzymes to "digest" lung tissue
2. Deficiency is either "heterozygous or homozygous"!

General

There is a series of genotypes called the "Pi" proteinase inhibitor system, characterized by isoelectric focusing and acid starch gel electrophoresis according to their mobilities. So far, there are eleven autosomal, codominant alleles recognized. They are labeled B, E, F, G, I, M, S, O, P, V, and Z, for a total of 121 possible phenotypes, eleven of which are homozygous and 110 of which are heterozygous, with MM being the most common. Only the ZZ Pi type has been unequivocally associated with pulmonary emphysema. The ZZ phenotype is also associated with cirrhosis, particularly juvenile cirrhosis. Patients with ZZ phenotype have been shown to have PAS-positive glycoprotein, which may be an abnormal alpha-1 antitrypsin inhibitor, in their hepatocytes.

Criteria

Pi phenotype	*MM*	*MZ*	*ZZ*
Level of antitrypsin	100%	61%	10%
Estimated frequency in general population	Over 90%	2–3%	1%
Risk of emphysema	"Normal" No increased risk	Increased incidence of emphysema with exposure to environmental factors	Develop emphysema even without exposure to environmental factors

Alpha-1-Antitrypsin Deficiency vs. Classic Emphysema

Criteria	ZZ Phenotype	MM Phenotype
Cases in women	High percentage	Very uncommon
Age	90% - under age 50 60% - under age 40	Most patients over age 50
Location	Most pronounced in lower lobes & panlobular	Generalized throughout lungs— centrilobular or panlobular
Exertional dyspnea preceded by chronic bronchitis	No	Usually

Note: Only about 5% of all emphysema patients have homozygous (ZZ) alpha-1 antitrypsin deficiency.

PULMONARY EMPHYSEMA CLASSIFICATION

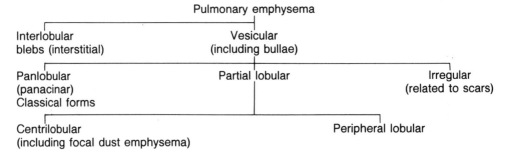

Pulmonary emphysema

Interlobular
blebs (interstitial)

Vesicular
(including bullae)

Panlobular
(panacinar)
Classical forms

Partial lobular

Irregular
(related to scars)

Centrilobular
(including focal dust emphysema)

Peripheral lobular

INTERSTITIAL EMPHYSEMA

Definition

Air outside NORMAL air spaces

Causes

Most common causes in adults:
a. spontaneous rupture of a bulla
b. 2nd most common, surgical or accidental tear
Most common causes in children:
a. overdistension due to artificial respiration
b. severe coughing, whooping cough, etc.

Key Words

Crepitant, sacs are blebs NOT bullae

Hamman's Syndrome

Spontaneous tear of lung with mediastinal emphysema and crushing pain mimicking myocardial infarct

Vesicular Emphysema

Type	Distensive	Destructive
Centrilobular		
Panlobular		
Paraseptal—peripheral lobular	(Functionally insignificant)	
Irregular or scar	(Most common at APEX of lungs)	

Major Types of Pulmonary Vesicular Emphysema

	Centrilobular	*Panlobular*	*Focal—Scar*
Location	Upper lobes, worse in central part of lobe	Usually occurs in patches in any lobe	Apex with TBC or anywhere
Obstruction	+	+	+
Alpha-1 antitrypsin defect	No	Some cases	No
Pigment	4+	+−	+−
Fibrous strands	+−to none in distensive; many *coarse* pigmented strands in destructive	4+ (fine strands) (Classically not pigmented)	3+
Capillary bed	Absent proximal vessels	Present but poorly functioning	Absent in scar
Incidence	60% of London emphysema cases		

Special comments	1. Distensive and destructive type
	2. ALWAYS PIGMENTED
	3. Pigment due to:
	   a. central migration of macrophages
	   b. poor blood supply and lymphatic (?) supply In centrilobular region
	4. Most common type of emphysema
	5. May have bullae
	6. Frequently have mixed panlobular and centrilobular emphysema
		1. Most common type to show bullae due to scar retraction
		2. Bullae most common on medial aspect of upper lobe
		3. Giant bullae-surgical emphysema
		4. Frequently occurs in areas of honeycombing, usually secondary to interstitial pneumonitis
			1. Puckering of pleura
			2. Scar carcinoma (adenocarcinoma) may occur, especially in nonapical scars

Instant Recognition of Patients With Emphysema

	Blue Bloater	*Pink Puffer*
Gross Emphysema	No	Yes
Clinical	Hypoventilate Polycythemia Cor pulmonale	Hyperventilate

(Continued on facing page)

Instant Recognition of Patients with Emphysema *(continued)*

	Blue Bloater	Pink Puffer
	Cyanosis, somnolence, and heart failure; obese, placid, happy person with fat face, low oxygen saturation, Pco_2 over 45	Thin, anxious person with thin face, near normal oxygen saturation, Pco_2 under 45
X-ray	Plethora of vessels	EMPHYSEMA
Pathology	1. Chronic obstructive bronchitis, out to pleura 2. Marked lack of emphysema 3. Squamous metaplasia, mucous gland metaplasia	1. Diffuse panlobular and/or centrilobular emphysema 2. Bullae often present
Key words	Cystic fibrosis, asthma, chronic bronchitis associated	May have alpha-1 antitrypsin defect

CLUBBING OF THE FINGERS

Definition

Edema and fibrous overgrowths of periosteal soft tissue at fingertips and toe tips, may be painful

Etiology and Pathogenesis

Basically unknown, but often associated with pulmonary disease and increased blood flow (?), estrogens, and other

DISEASES COMMONLY ASSOCIATED WITH CLUBBING OF FINGERS
(Note: When underlying disease is cured, clubbing disappears.)

Pulmonary

1. Bronchogenic carcinoma, about 5% show clubbing
2. Chronic lung infections, abscess, bronchiectasis, (clubbing rare with TBC)
3. Emphysema
4. Pleural mesothelioma (50% of cases show clubbing)

Cardiovascular

1. Any congenital heart disease, especially those with cyanosis (right-to-left shunt)
2. Subacute bacterial endocarditis

Hepatic

1. Cirrhosis, especially biliary cirrhosis

Gastrointestinal

1. Ulcerative colitis, regional enteritis
2. Malabsorption syndromes

Neoplasms

Especially chronic granulocytic leukemia

6 Congenital Heart Diseases

Intraventricular Septal Defect	Intra-atrial Defect	Lutembacher's Disease

Clinical

1. Loud systolic machinery murmur 2. Precordial thrill 3. Cyanosis late 4. Survival depends on *size* of defect	1. Loud systolic murmur 2. Sx depend on *size* of lesion 3. Cyanosis late	1. Atrial septal defect, usually large 2. Mitral stenosis 3. Cyanosis late 4. More common in females

Pathology

1. Membranous anterior defect most common 2. Muscular defect least common but worse prognosis 3. Cor triloculare biatriatum is extreme form—frogs 4. Jet lesion, Zahn-Schminke pockets common 5. Get RVH and pulmonary stenosis late 6. SBE is a complication in up to 40% of cases	1. *Type I,* ostium primum defect: lack of cardiac cushion development; defect LOW, usually large; poorer prognosis 2. *Type II,* ostium secundum defect: lack of competent closure of foramen ovale; high, usually small; better prognosis 3. Get RVH and pulmonary stenosis late 4. Cor triloculare biventriculare is extreme form	1. IASD primum or secundum 2. Mitral stenosis, congenital or acquired (rheumatic usually) 3. Atrial dilation, bilateral 4. RVH (NO LVH)

Key Words

1. *Most common* (25% of all CHD cases) clinically significant congenital anomaly of the heart 2. Cyanotic late with R-to-L shunt 3. Average survival, 14.5 years	1. Most common, but usually nonsymptomatic defect, patent (by probe) foramen ovale, in 25% of adults 2. Secondary membrane grows to right of ostium primum 3. Cyanotic late with R-to-L shunt 4. Prognosis poor with septum primum, good with septum secundum	1. 5% of all ASD cases have mitral stenosis 2. Rarely live past age 35

Transposition of Great Vessels vs. Taussig-Bing Complex

Transposition of Great Vessels		*Taussig-Bing Complex*
Uncorrected	Corrected	
1. Only aorta and pulmonary arteries transposed	1. Right and left sides of heart are MIRROR IMAGES	1. Rare
2. Much more common than corrected	2. Aorta, coronary arteries, LV muscle patterns and mitral valve in "right" (ANTERIOR) ventricle	2. Aorta arises from RV
3. Must have patent abnormal opening between pulmonary and systemic circuits for survival	3. Pulmonary artery, RV muscle patterns and tricuspid valve, "left" (POSTERIOR) ventricle	3. With pulmonary artery overriding IVSD
4. Prognosis POOR	4. Venous return also mirrored	4. Get RVH
	5. No symptoms if no other anomaly present	5. Differentiated from Eisenmenger complex by:
	6. About 50% of cases have other significant anomalies	a. oxygen saturation in pulmonary artery greater than in right atrium
	7. Prognosis better than uncorrected	b. early cyanosis

Tetralogy of Fallot vs. Eisenmenger Complex

	Tetralogy of Fallot	*Eisenmenger Complex*
IVSD	Yes	Yes
RVH	Yes	Yes
Overriding aorta	Yes	Yes
Pulmonary stenosis	Yes (usually infundibular)	No
Key words	1. Patent ductus arteriosus common (pentalogy)	1. Rarer than tetralogy
	2. Most common cause of cyanotic heart disease	2. Pulmonary hypertension present, Cyanosis less severe than tetralogy
	3. Clinical:	3. Average survival = 25 years
	a. early cyanosis and polycythemia	
	b. clubbing of fingers	
	c. squatting	
	d. systolic murmur and thrill over chest	
	e. emboli and SBE are common complications	
	4. Average survival = 12 years	

PATENT DUCTUS ARTERIOSUS

1. 80% closed by 3 months; all close by 2 years if normal
2. Machinery murmur and systolic thrill; Corrigan's pulse
3. No cyanosis until late with right-to-left shunt. Average age of survival = 40 years
4. More common in females (3:1)

COARCTATION OF AORTA

Adult Type

1. Postductal location
2. Death usually by age 40
3. Death due to:
   a. CHF
   b. emboli
   c. rupture of dissecting (medionecrosis) aneurysm, 25% of cases
   d. CVA (hypertension)
4. Clinical
   a. rib notching
   b. hypertension in upper extremities
   c. "red outs"
   d. systolic murmur
5. 40% have bicuspid aortic valve

Infantile Type

1. Preductal location
2. Death soon after birth
3. Most blood flows through ductus; obliterative endoarteritis of proximal aorta

EBSTEIN'S MALFORMATION

1. Rare
2. Posterior and downward displacement of dorsal leaflets of tricuspid valve
3. *NOT* the same as tricuspid atresia

CHIARI'S NETWORK

1. Rare
2. Threadlike meshwork of bands in right atrium
3. Can be associated with bacterial endocarditis and thrombi in right atrium

7 Arteriosclerosis–Newer Concepts

TAKE HOME MESSAGE ABOUT ATHEROSCLEROSIS

1. There are several theories about the etiology of arteriosclerosis
2. The disease is probably one of multiple etiologies. (See table of risk factors on page 45)
3. The theory currently held by most researchers in the field, based on human and experimental studies, is the lipid theory

MYTHS ABOUT ARTERIOSCLEROSIS

1. Hypertension causes increased arteriosclerosis
    a. much hypertension in African natives, almost NO arteriosclerosis
    b. most patients dying of myocardial infarcts have small or normal-sized hearts
    c. much more hypertension, but 1/3 fewer infarcts in American blacks than in whites
2. Obesity causes increased arteriosclerosis
    Most pateints with myocardial infarcts are NOT obese

THEORIES OF ETIOLOGY OF ATHEROSCLEROSIS

Thrombogenic Theory

Lesion due to a thrombus on arterial wall with organization, endothelialization, and degeneration

Rokitansky—19th century
Duguid—20th century England

Intramural Hemorrhage Theory

More vasa vasorum in areas of plaques, intramural hemorrhage seen, but late

Winternitz—Yale 1938

Lipid Theory

Lipid theory based on:
a. plasma lipid studies, humans and animals
    1. congenital hyperlipidemias—Fredrickson 1967
    2. acquired hyperlipidemias
b. geographic studies
    1. high atherosclerosis as in advanced countries with high-fat diets
    2. low, as in underdeveloped countries with low-fat diets
c. experimental animal studies
    1. no arteriosclerosis with low-fat diets
    2. much arteriosclerosis with high-fat diets, MINI PIGS are most like humans

Stamler—1952; Keys—1957; Sisson and Thomas—1968

FACTS SUPPORTING LIPID THEORY

1. High-fat diets associated with more arteriosclerosis than low fat diets
   High relative percentage saturated fatty acids and high level of cholesterol are worst
2. The following plasma lipids are associated with arteriosclerosis:
   a. cholesterol (free and esters)
   b. triglycerides
   c. β-lipoproteins
   d. saturated fatty acids; high unsaturated fat diet may cause cancer
   e. free fatty acid (NEFA) in acute myocardial infarction
3. Abnormal coagulation of blood has been seen in animals and humans on a high fat diet
   a. elevated fibrinogen
   b. elevated prothrombin levels (shortened prothrombin time)
   c. prolonged clot lysis time (plasmin system inhibition)
   d. prolonged euglobulin lysis time
   e. stronger clots (more cross-linkages—amide, S-S ?)

DEVELOPMENT OF ATHEROSCLEROTIC LESION (Experimental Mini Pigs)

Preproliferative Phase

1. Imbibition of cholesterol-rich fluid into extracellular and intracellular compartments of arterial wall
2. Lipids in plaques have pattern of serum, not tissue, fatty acids; (e.g. linoleate)
3. Damage and occasional death of scattered endothelial and smooth-muscle cells (SMC), usually in small clusters in inner wall
4. Foci of formed and nonformed elements of blood seen in intimal extracellular compartment
5. Increased turnover rate (T3 thymidine) of endothelial and SMC to replace damaged cells and/or as a result of direct stimulation

Proliferative Phase

1. Focal proliferation of SMC to exceed replacement needs producing small masses in intima and inner media. SMC in each plaque monoclonal by G-6-PD testing
2. Cycle of damage and excessive proliferation proceeds at variable pace in above masses
3. *First grossly visible lesions* occur at this stage
4. Ghost bodies (membrane-bound granular bodies, thought to be degenerated portions of RER of SMC) first appear
5. Foam cells first appear in this phase; they are either:
   a. macrophages filled with fat, or
   b. SMC filled with fat
6. Fate of SMC (myofilaments):
   a. degenerate (ghost bodies)
   b. imbibe fat (foam cells)
   c. become fibroblasts, lots of RER (collagen fibrils), most common in late proliferative phase and atheromatous phase, A SCAR IS A SCAR. Lipids in fibrous plaques have tissue pattern (e.g. high oleate)

Atheromatous Phase

1. Larger foci of dead cells appear (necrosis) resulting in beginning of an atheroma
2. Foci increase in number and coalesce, making larger masses of necrotic debris
3. In areas of necrosis, cholesterol (imbibed and released) precipitates and crystallizes as do other substances, such as calcium

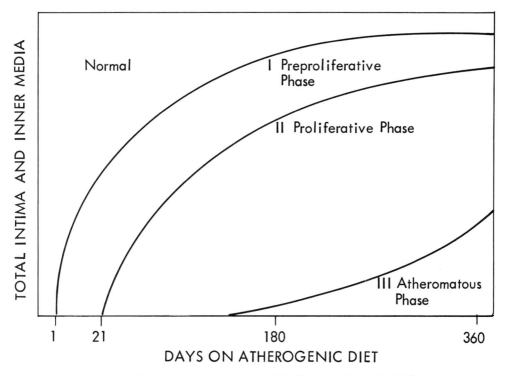

Fig. 7–1. Development of atherosclerotic lesion (experimental mini pigs).

Notes

1. Thrombosis may be superimposed on atheromatous plaque
2. Get increased vasa vasorum underlying atheromatous lesion, may get hemorrhage into plaques
3. Aortic atherosclerosis most severe in abdominal aorta
4. Coronary arteries: most severe in anterior descending branch of left coronary artery with occlusion in the 1st 2 centimeters, final occlusion most commonly due to thrombus superimposed on atheromatous plaque

ANOXIC INJURY OF THE MYOCARDIUM

Understanding of this section presupposes a *working* knowledge of NORMAL myocardial anatomy, physiology and biochemistry. Please review in the appropriate texts.

General

1. Normally anaerobic metabolism accounts for 1% of total energy of the myocardium; during hypoxia, this is about 10%, but is inadequate
2. 20% of deaths of Caucasians in the U.S.A. are due to acute myocardial infarction
3. Myocardial damage due to ischemia is reversible up to 18 minutes (point of no return), after this NO

MYOCARDIAL INFARCTS

Myocardial Changes With Ischemia

Time of Infarction	Changes
Prenecrotic Phase	
20–30 minutes	Loss of oxidative phosphorylation, electron transport, and sodium pump. Swelling of mitochondria and RER with disaggregation of ribosomes (EM)
60 minutes	Mitochondria: swollen, increased calcium, intramatrixial granules, calcium phosphate causes uncoupling

I Bands: prominent (relaxation of myofibrils)
Glycogen granules: decreased or absent
Nuclear chromatin: margination
ER: swollen, expanded cisternae
Membranes: increased permeability and inability to regulate ion fluxes
Ion fluxes continue:
OUT: K^+, Mg^{++}, Cl^-
IN: Na^+, Ca^{++}
Lysosomes: lyse with lowered pH due to excess lactate release; acid phosphatase, cathepsins, DNAase, RNAase, β glucuronidase, α maltase, and others

Necrotic Phase	
8–12 hours	First changes visible by light microscope; eosinophilia of myocardial cytoplasm and loss of cross striations
24 hours	Pyknosis, karyolysis, karyorrhexis, swollen granular eosinophilic cytoplasm, polys begin to arrive, acute pericarditis begins, healed in 4 weeks
48–72 hours	Polys peak and start to lyse, all gone by Day 14; mononuclear cells begin to phagocytose fat and dead cells
Day 4 to Day 11	Granulation tissue begins to grow in, macrophages take away debris, mural thrombi may occur, organized by Day 16
Healing Phase	
Day 12	Collagen first appears, prominent at 3 weeks and maximal at 2 months; contraction begins at 6 weeks
3 weeks	Prominent collagen
6 weeks	Collagen begins to contract
8 weeks	A SCAR IS A SCAR IS A SCAR

COMPLICATIONS OF MYOCARDIAL INFARCTS

1. Cardiac arrhythmias: probably most common cause of death in *ACUTE* MI
2. Congestive heart failure: 20% of MI patients have CHF. Causes 30 to 40% of MI deaths
3. Mural thrombus: 20–25% of MI patients; may give thromboemboli
4. Cardiogenic shock: 10% of MI patients
5. Cardiac aneurysm: 5% to 10%; very few rupture
6. Myocardial rupture with tamponade: 5% of MI patients, most common 5th to 10th day

PROGNOSIS OF MYOCARDIAL INFARCT

Acute (die in less than 2 weeks)

Overall acute MI mortality: 12%
With *NO* shock, CHF or serious arrhythmia: 0%
With *ONE* of the signs (shock, CHF, or serious arrhythmia): 17%
With *TWO* or more of the signs (shock, CHF, or serious arrhythmia): 57%

Overall MI mortality rate, acute and chronic

75% in 10 years
50% in 5 years
25% in 6 weeks

FACTORS CURRENTLY RECOGNIZED TO INCREASE RISK OF MYOCARDIAL INFARCTS

1. High fat diet
2. Hyperlipidemia
3. Hypertension
4. Obesity
5. Cigarette smoking
6. Soft water
7. Age
8. Sex
9. Physical activity
10. Heredity
11. Emotional stress (type A behavioral pattern)
12. Diabetes

8 Valvular Heart Diseases

	Rheumatic Heart Disease	Syphilitic Heart Disease
Incidence	3rd most common heart disease	Less than 1% of heart disease
Etiology	Group A beta-hemolytic strep, probably abnormal immunity	*Treponema pallidum*
Clinical	Usually in children Major manifestations a. Migratory polyarthritis (85%) b. Carditis (65%) c. Sydenham's chorea (30%) d. Erythema marginatum e. Subcutaneous nodules	Usually in middle age A form of tertiary syphilis Tambour murmur Corrigan-wide pulse

Pathology	*Cardiac involvement*
	1. *Endocardium*
	  a. mitral valve (40%)
	    1) short, thick chordae tendineae
	  b. aortic and mitral together (35%–40%)
	  c. aortic valve alone (15%)
	    1) thick, rolled leaflets
	    2) fusion of commissures
	  d. Vegetations (acute) small (1–2 mm. diameter); on line of closure; NO bacteria or fibrin; fibrosis late (?)
	  e. (Chronic) MacCallum patch, left atrium
	2. *Myocardium*
	(Fibrin to Aschoff bodies to scar)
	Aschoff bodies—Aschoff giant cells, Anitschkow myocytes (owl-eye, caterpillar), lymphs, plasma cells, fibroblasts
	3. *Pericardium*
	Fibrin, bread-and-butter pericarditis
		Valvular involvement
		(Primarily aortic valve)
		Spreading of commissures, thickening and rolling of cusps
		
		Aorta
		Gross:
		1. Tree-barking
		2. Stellate scars
		
		Micro:
		1. Perivascular cuffing: lymphocytes and plasma cells around small vessels; vasa vasorum with obliterative endarteritis
		2. Primary lesion, destruction of aortic elastica by (?)spirochetes or anoxia
		Levaditi silver stain for spirochetes

(Continued on facing page)

(continued)

	Rheumatic Heart Disease	Syphilitic Heart Disease
Complications	Arrhythmias, cardiac failure, interstitial pneumonitis, predisposition to SBE, and embolization, especially from atrial mural thrombi	Aortic insufficiency (Zahn-Schmincke pockets) Aortic aneurysm (ascending aorta), tracheal tug, hoarseness, brassy cough, may rupture Coronary insufficiency, very rare

Bacterial (Vegetative) Endocarditis

	Acute (ABE)	Subacute (SBE)
Duration	Less than 50 days	More than 50 days
Valve	Often previously normal	Usually previously diseased (RHD and congenital)
Organism	More virulent	Less virulent
Pre-antibiotic era	Staphylococcus Beta-hemolytic strep	Alpha-hemolytic streptococcus (*Strep. viridans* 75%)
Post-antibiotic era	Staphylococcus Fungi	Strep viridans (less than 50%) Staph, fungi, gram-negative organisms (increasing as cause)
Clinical	Splinter hemorrhages (Osler's nodes) under nails, murmurs, hematuria, splenomegaly	
Vegetations	Largest (1–2 cm.) vegetations, friable (usually 1 or 2 in number) and on free margin of valve; sometimes extend behind valve leaflet	
Location	Mitral most common (75%) Mitral and aortic (60%) Right side valves, (15%) tricuspid more than pulmonic	
Micro	Fibrin, amorphous material, bacteria, red cells, few white cells; to fibrosis if heals Vascularized underlying leaflet	
Complications	1. Focal embolic glomerulonephritis (hematuria); no organisms in the glomeruli 2. Splinter hemorrhages under nails (Osler's nodes) 3. Petechiae on skin 4. Myocardial microabscesses (Bracht-Wachter bodies) rare 5. Brain and other abscesses, infarcts due to emboli	

Cardiac Valvular Vegetations

	Marantic Endocarditis	Libman-Sacks Endocarditis	Carcinoid Heart Disease
Location and size of vegetation	1. Usually occur on line of closure, but can occur elsewhere 2. Most common on mitral valve (uncommon elsewhere) 3. 1–5 mm. diameter 4. Usually multiple	1. Random location on valve 2. Usually on mitral and tricuspid valves 3. Usually small (1–3 mm.) diameter 4. Usually multiple	1. Exclusively on right side of heart 2. Most common on tricuspid valve 3. Mast cells and amorphous material progressing to fibrosis late 4. Later get fibrosis above internal elastic lamina with endocardial thickening, may get tricuspid and pulmonic stenosis and RVH
Special features	1. Also called nonbacterial thrombotic endocarditis 2. Micro: amorphous to fibrin with no significant inflammation 3. In patients with debilitating diseases (cancer, etc.) 4. Can become emboli with infarcts of brain, kidney, spleen, etc. 5. May be related to a hypercoagulable state	1. Also called nonbacterial verrucous endocarditis 2. Seen in 55% of lupus erythematosus cases 3. Amorphous: fibrinoid-fibrin 4. May have hematoxylin bodies, some inflammatory cells 5. Also commonly have diffuse fibrinous pericarditis	1. Part of carcinoid syndrome 2. Carcinoid syndrome a. flushing, blushing, diarrhea, bronchoconstriction b. due to excess serotonin 3. Must have hepatic metastases (never from appendix) 4. Serotonin detoxified in lung by MAO 5. Diagnosis by HIAA in urine

9 Pericarditis and Miscellaneous Heart Diseases

Endocardial Thickenings

Disease or Associated Condition	Type of Thickening	Key Words
Zahn-Schmincke pockets (jet lesion)	Fibrosis + capillaries (no elastica)	1. MOST common in left ventricle; associated with aortic insufficiency 2. Convexity in direction of regurgitation
Hypertension	Relative thickening: *all* layers of endocardium, intima, smooth muscle, elastica	1. MOST common in left ventricle 2. USUALLY focal
Organized thrombus; healed myocardial infarct	Fibrous (scar) (collagen) Hyaline	USUALLY focal subendocardial infarct
Indwelling catheter or pacemaker	Pure elastica	1. Inert foreign body (?) 2. Focal
Endocardial fibroelastosis	Mostly collagen and elastica with some smooth muscle	1. MOST common in children 2. MOST common in left ventricle 3. USUALLY diffuse, both inflow and outflow tracts 4. Globular 5. (?) Etiology: congenital, intrauterine anoxia or inflammation 6. Other congenital anomalies common
Endomyocardial fibrosis	Fibrin to fibrous thickening with some smooth muscle proliferation extending into subendocardial myocardium (no elastica)	1. MOST common in children (Africa) 2. MOST common in inflow tract of left ventricle 3. NEVER in outflow tract 4. Contracted heart with point at apex

(Continued on overleaf)

Endocardial Thickenings (continued)

Disease or Associated Condition	Type of Thickening	Key Words
Becker's heart disease	Early—acute inflammation with bland infarcts and emboli Late—fibroelastica thickening, focal	1. Common in South Africa 2. Also a subendocardial cardiomyopathy Early: acute inflammation with bland infarcts 3. Thickened subendocardial arteries with verrucous angiitis
Loffler's endocarditis	Early: fibrinous focal lesions on endocardium Late: fibrosis, diffuse, of endocardium with some elastica	1. Left ventricle MOST common 2. Eosinophilic arteritis 3. Eosinophilic infiltrations, subendocardial and endocardial

Congenital Cardiomyopathies

	Key Lesion	Special Features
Familial cardiomyopathy	Focal degeneration of myocardial fibers to scars	1. Familial history, over several generations 2. *RARE*
Hurler's cardiomyopathy	Abnormal lysosomes in histiocytes and muscle cells (dermatan and heparitin sulfate)	1. Gargoylism, lysosomal disease—lack of alpha-L-iduronidase 2. Generalized abnormal mucopolysaccharide metabolism
Friedreich's ataxia cardiomyopathy	Ventricular hypertrophy Degeneration and vacuolation of myocardial cells with foci of chronic inflammatory cells	Also degeneration of posterior columns, corticospinal and dorsal spinocerebellar tracts

Infectious Cardiomyopathies

Diphtheritic cardiomyopathy	Early: cellular hyaline and fatty degeneration with neutrophils Late: chronic inflammatory cells + SCAR	1. May also have endocarditis 2. MOST common cause of death in diphtheria 3. Due to toxin, NO bacteria in heart
Viral cardiomyopathy	Focal degerneration of fibers; lymphocytes + plasma cells, later scar	1. Coxsackie B MOST common known virus Almost any virus can cause 2. Hard to prove etiology
Chagas' cardiomyopathy	Unwinding of myocardial fiber bundles Eosinophils focally with degenerated cells, later scarring	1. Part of generalized Chagas' disease 2. MOST common cause of sudden death in South America 3. *Trypanosoma cruzi* usually in ganglion cells and cardiac cells
Other infections: rickettsia, trichinella, fungi	Focal infectious organisms often seen	*Trichinella spiralis* does not encyst in heart

Metabolic and Toxic Cardiomyopathies

Pompe's disease (Type II glycogen storage disease)	Large vacuolated cells, PAS-positive, glycogen in lysosomes	1. Glycogen storage disease 2. Lack of lysosomal maltase 3. Heart also involved in Types III and IV glycogen storage disease
Myxedema cardiomyopathy	Swelling of muscle fibers Interstitial mucoid material	1. Hypothyroid, T4 low 2. Part of generalized myxedema
Amyloid heart disease	Collections of amyloid between myocardial cells	Almost always associated with primary amyloidosis
Hypokalemia	Nonspecific foci of inflammatory cells	EKG changes: flat T waves
Chloroform, phosphorus	Fatty and vacuolar degeneration of myocardial cells to scar	Often die in acute heart failure

Nutritional and Idiopathic Cardiomyopathies

Beriberi cardiomyopathy	Dilated, flabby heart May have cloudy swelling + fatty degeneration of muscle cells	1. Thiamine deficiency 2. Part of WET beriberi 3. Found in some alcoholics
Alcoholic cardiomyopathy	Similar to beriberi above, but also have mural thrombi and patchy fibrosis	1. No thiamine deficiency 2. ? direct toxic effect of alcohol on myocardium
Beer drinker's cardiomyopathy	EM: mitochondrial and E. R. swelling Foci of degenerated heart cells; later focal scar	1. Due to cobalt in beer as an antifoam agent 2. Cobalt *NOT* in beer now
Sarcoid cardiomyopathy	Sarcoid granulomas	1. 20% of sarcoids involve heart 2. 2/3 of cases have sudden death 3. Arrhythmias common
Collagen diseases	Foci of fibrosis and vasculitis	Part of generalized syndromes
Fiedler's cardiomyopathy (idiopathic)	Histology variable, focal acute and/or chronic cells; later scar	Diagnose only after ruling out those of known etiology (wastebasket diagnosis ?)

PERICARDITIS

Acute Fibrinous and Serous Pericarditis

Disease or Associated Condition	Key Lesion	Special Features
Uremia	Fibrin, diffuse	1. MOST common cause of generalized fibrinous pericarditis in U. S. A. 2. High BUN 3. Part of generalized uremia
Myocardial infarct	Fibrin, focal over infarct	MOST common cause of focal fibrinous pericarditis in U.S.A.
Rheumatic pericarditis	Acute, classic bread-and-butter pericarditis	1. MOST common cause of fibrinous pericarditis in children in U. S. A. 2. Decreasing in incidence 3. Part of generalized acute RHD
Congestive heart failure (serous pericarditis)	Clear, watery fluid; resolves without scar	1. MOST common cause of serous pericarditis 2. Also have hydrothorax and ascites
Concato's disease	Generalized polyserositis	1. Can get constrictive pericarditis if severe 2. Part of generalized serositis

Hemorrhagic Pericarditis

MOST common causes (in order of frequency):
1. Tuberculosis
2. Malignant tumors
   a. lung
   b. breast
   c. melanoma
   d. lymphoma

Hemopericardium

MOST common causes (in order of frequency):
1. Trauma to heart
2. Myocardial infarct with rupture (5% of myocardial infarcts)
3. Dissecting aneurysm of aorta

Constrictive Pericarditis

MOST common causes (in order of frequency):
1. Idiopathic (no etiologic agent found)
2. Tuberculous pericarditis
3. Staphylococcal pericarditis

Key Words: Small, quiet heart

Special Syndrome: Pick's disease 1. Constrictive pericarditis. 2. Compression of vena cava.

10 Miscellaneous Vascular Diseases

Nonatherosclerotic Arterial Disease I

	Monckeberg's Medial Sclerosis	Buerger's Disease (Thromboangiitis Obliterans)	Pulseless Disease (Takayasu's Syndrome)
Clinical	1. Male = female incidence 2. Calcification, common over 50 years on x-ray 3. Lower extremity arteries MOST common, also coronary arteries 4. NO symptoms	1. Young males, usually Jews 2. Associated with smoking 3. May or may not show atherosclerosis 4. Both upper and lower extremity involved 5. May have great pain	1. Women to men = 9:1 2. USUALLY under 50 years old 3. Weak pulses in upper extremity, visual disturbances, reverse coarctation
Gross	1. Hard, calcified nodularity 2. Gooseneck-lamp nodularity	Focal vascular occlusion	1. Narrow lumen and occluded aortic arch and branches 2. Thick-walled aorta
Micro	1. Medial calcification 2. Basophilic degeneration 3. NO intimal involvement	1. Acute to chronic inflammation and microabscesses 2. Thrombi with recanalization 3. Phlebitis and neuritis also seen	1. Adventitial fibrosis, medial fibrosis 2. Perivascular lymphocytes and plasma cells 3. Superimposed atherosclerosis and thrombosis may occur
Key words	1. Etiology unknown 2. Is arteriosclerosis but NOT atherosclerosis 3. Involves medium-sized arteries 4. May predispose to atherosclerosis	1. Extends to involve veins and nerves as well as arteries 2. May be an accelerated form (galloping) of atherosclerosis	Etiology unknown a. special type of atherosclerosis b. allergic vasculitis

Nonatherosclerotic Arterial Disease II

	Temporal Arteritis (Giant Cell Arteritis)	Rheumatoid Arteritis	Cystic Medionecrosis of Erdheim
Clinical	Males = females; over 50 years old usually; Throbbing pain over arterial areas USUALLY self-limiting, but may become generalized in 10%–15% of cases	Rheumatoid arthritis, often juvenile, with aortitis, arteritis, with or without cardiac symptoms	Male 3 : female 1, congenital Peak age over 50 years Often associated with Marfan's syndrome Hypertension frequently associated Dissecting aneurysm is sequela; may mimic MI (more back pain ?)
Gross	Nodular swelling over arteries	Aorta most commonly involved, also may involve medium-sized and smaller arteries	Transverse intimal tear in ascending aorta in 95% (in 5% no tear found) Dissection between inner 2/3 and outer 1/3 of media
Micro	Starts in intima and progresses to all layers Neutrophils to eosinophils to mononuclear cells, often have giant cell granulomas May have thrombi All layers involved in classic lesion	Looks much like luetic aortitis: perivascular lymphocytes and plasma cells Acutely, may look like other collagen vasculitides with neutrophils	Cysts (cystic degeneration) Mucoid degeneration; acid mucopolysaccharides; alcian green stain Elastica degeneration
Special features	May become generalized and involve aorta + coronary arteries; giant cell aortitis Etiology unknown, allergic (?) vasculitis Blindness is MOST common serious complication	55% of rheumatoid arthritis cases have some cardiovascular involvement May have myocardial infarct	Hemopericardium and double-barrel aorta common May get secondary myocardial infarct with coronary occlusion Produced in animals with beta-aminoproprionitrile from sweet peas (lathyrism)

Benign Tumors of Blood Vessels

Disease	Key Words
Capillary hemangioma	1. Most common on skin; also seen in internal viscera 2. Port wine nevus is an example
Cavernous hemangioma	1. Most common benign tumor of liver 2. Sinusoids and larger vascular channels 3. Malignancy very rare
von Hippel-Lindau disease	1. Cavernous hemangioma involving: cerebellum, eye grounds, pancreas and liver
Sclerosing hemangioma (dermatofibroma)	1. Most common in skin 2. Pigmented brown nonencapsulated lesion with occluded vascular channels, fibrosis, hemosiderin-laden macrophages, and occasional giant cells 3. No malignant potential
Glomangioma	1. Very painful 2. Most common on fingertips and under nails 3. Composed of blood vessels and nests of glomus cells 4. Function of glomus body—regulation of arterial flow
Hemangiopericytoma	1. Rare tumor of pericytes (smooth muscle cells) outside arterial basement membrane of blood vessels 2. Micro: organoid, around vessels 3. Looks benign, but up to 50% metastasize
Carotid body tumor	1. Tumor causes hypotension on manipulation 2. Micro: aggregates of epithelioid cells ("Zellballen") 3. Malignancy very rare
Hemangioendothelioma	1. Benign tumor of endothelial cells 2. Must differentiate from hemangioma, granulation tissue, and hemangiosarcoma

Malignant Tumor of Blood Vessels

Hemangioendotheliosarcoma (angiosarcoma)	1. Very rare in general population 2. Most commonly seen in skin; also liver and spleen 3. Industrial exposure to vinyl chloride monomer associated with high incidence in liver 4. Micro: masses of malignant endothelial cells with abortive blood vessel formation

Nontumorous Lymphatic Diseases

	Lymphedema Praecox	*Milroy's Disease*	*Simple Congenital Lymphedema*
Clinical	MOST common in pubertal females	1. Lymphedema present from birth 2. Many relatives with syndrome	1. Present from birth 2. No family history
Gross	1. Edema of feet, progressing to legs, thighs, etc. 2. Dilated lymphatics; may lead to secondary skin changes	Confined almost entirely to lower extremities	Otherwise same as Milroy's disease
Micro	Dilated lymphatics with slight inflammation (nonspecific)	Fibrosis + scarring around lymphatics due to long-standing edema	
Special features	1. Etiology unknown 2. Uncommon disease	1. Faulty (?) development of lymphatics 2. Other forms may involve face, arms independently	

Tumors of Lymphatics: Key Words

Lymphangioma	*Lymphangiosarcoma*	*Cavernous Lymphangioma (Cystic Hygroma)*
1. Uncommon 2. Most common around neck and axilla 3. Usually under 2 cm. diameter 4. Differentiate from hemangiomas by lack of RBC's in channels 5. Malignancy very rare	1. Very rare 2. Seen ONLY in axilla after radical mastectomy	1. Most common in children 2. Most common in neck and axilla 3. Usually large, up to 15 cm. diameter 4. Most important because of: disfigurement and obstruction of airway, foodway and blood vessels in neck 5. Malignancy very rare

DISEASES OF VEINS

Superior Vena Cava Obstruction (Syndrome)

1. Tumor MOST common cause
2. Bronchogenic carcinoma is MOST common tumor to cause
3. Also inflammation and thrombi may occlude

Inferior Vena Cava Obstruction (Syndrome)

1. MOST common is propagation of clot from iliac vein
2. Second most common is renal cell carcinoma in vena cava

Portal Vein Thrombosis

Usually associated with cirrhosis

Pyleophlebitis

1. Acute appendicitis MOST common cause
2. Also associated with acute cholecystitis and peritonitis

Mondor's Disease (String Phlebitis)

1. Thrombophlebitis of thoracoepigastric vein
2. May be mistaken for metastatic tumor, usually breast

Veno-occlusive Disease (Intrahepatic Venous Occlusion)

Associated with "bush"-tea drinkers in Jamaica

Phlegmasia Alba Dolens (Milk Leg)

1. MOST common in lower extremity postpartum
2. Commonly painful

TELANGIECTASIA

Spider Telangiectasia

1. Associated with high estrogen levels
2. MOST common in upper portions of body in cirrhosis and pregnancy
3. Micro: dilated vessels

Rendu-Osler-Weber Disease (Hereditary Telangiectasia)

1. Dominant heredity, males and females equally
2. Present from birth
3. Micro: multiple small focal capillaries
4. Multiple aneurysmal telangiectases involving skin, GI, GU + respiratory systems
5. Bleeding may be fatal

Sturge-Weber Disease (Encephalotrigeminal Angiomatosis)

1. Hereditary, abnormal venous development, RARE
2. Syndrome consists of:
   a. port wine nevus of one side of face
   b. ipsilateral angiomatous masses in leptomeninges and cortical angiomatosis
   c. often associated with mental retardation

11 Oral Cavity and Salivary Glands

The Oral Cavity as a Mirror

Oral Disease	Associated Condition
Enamel discoloration	
1. Green-brown	Bile, erythroblastosis fetalis
2. Red	Congenital porphyria, uroporphyrin
3. Yellow-brown	Tetracycline therapy
4. Any color	Food and pigment-producing factors most common cause of enamel discoloration
Mottled enamel	Fluorine (more than 1.5 ppm) in drinking water
Koplik spots	Measles
Pregnancy tumor	1. Pregnancy, focal granuloma
	2. Occurs in about 20% of pregnancies
	3. Usually disappears after delivery
Lead line	1. Lead poisoning
	2. Pigmentation of gums, lead line
	3. Also seen with other heavy metals
Generalized hyperplasia of gingiva	1. Dilantin therapy for epilepsy
	2. Leukemia, especially monocytic type, leukemic cell infiltrates
Loss of lamina dura of teeth (x-ray)	Hyperparathyroidism
Generalized oral pigmentation	1. Peutz-Jeghers syndrome
	2. Addison's disease
	3. Argyria
Hutchinson's incisors Mulberry molars	Congenital syphilis
Periodontal disease, abscesses	1. Diabetes mellitus
	2. Micro: small vessel disease
Red-purple telangiectasia	Osler-Weber-Rendu

MISCELLANEOUS DISEASES OF THE ORAL CAVITY: KEY WORDS

Fordyce's Granules (Fordyce's Disease)

1. Ectopic sebaceous glands in buccal mucosa
2. No pathological significance

Epulis

1. Definition: tumor-like mass of gingiva
2. Most are reparative granulomas with prominent giant cell component
3. Most are cured with curettage
4. Rarely malignant

Dental Caries (Cavities)

1. Definition: chronic localized destructive disease of posteruptive teeth
2. Exact etiology unknown; suspect *Strep. mutans* and *sanguis*
3. The most common cause of tooth loss before age 45

Pyorrhea (Periodontitis)

1. Definition: acute-chronic inflammation around teeth
2. Most common cause for tooth loss after age 45
3. No pain
4. No generalized disease

Gingivitis

1. Definition: an inflammation, usually painless, (acute, subacute, or chronic) confined to the gingivae,
2. Etiology: bacteria, especially those in plaque on teeth surfaces
3. The most common disease of the mucous membranes

Trench Mouth (Vincent's Angina)

1. Definition: acute necrotizing inflammation of gingivae around teeth
2. Spirochetal, *Borrelia vincentii*
3. Very painful
4. May become a generalized lesion

Ranula

1. Definition: epithelial cyst in floor of mouth
2. From minor salivary glands (?)

Branchial Cleft Cyst

1. Embryonic remnant from third branchial cleft (mass in lateral neck)
2. With fistula, have opening at angle of jaw
3. MICRO: lined with epithelium, much lymphoid tissue around fistula

Thyroglossal Duct Cyst

1. Definition: cystic dilatation of thyroglossal duct which passes from foramen cecum (at base of tongue) to thyroid isthmus
2. Cystic enlargement in MIDLINE lined by columnar epithelium

Some Tumors of the Oral Cavity

	Ameloblastoma (Adamantinoma)	*Granular Cell Myoblastoma*
Clinical	Swollen jaw with destruction of bone	Small benign tumor
Location	Usually in mandible Most common extraoral location is pituitary (Rathke's pouch tumor) 2nd most common extraoral location is tibia	Tongue (35%) Skin and subcutaneous tissue, usually in breast (60%) Striated muscle and elsewhere (5%)
Pathology		
Micro	Islands of palisaded epithelium resembling enamel organ around central "star cells" with loose connective tissue stroma	Large polygonal cells with granular cytoplasm, no cross striations Contain lipoprotein and mucoprotein but *not* sudanophilic
Gross	Tumor, cystic mass, often large	Small (1–3 mm.), circumscribed but not encapsulated

Special features	1. Tumor of enamel organ
	2. Malignant potential doubtful "intermediate tumor"
	3. More common in females than males
		1. Origin NOT clear
		    muscle cells (?)
		    Schwann cells (?)
		    histiocytes (?)
		    xanthoma (?)
		2. Pseudoepitheliomatous hyperplasia of overlying epithelium often mistaken for cancer
		3. No malignant potential

Squamous Cell Carcinoma of Oral Cavity

Location	*Lower Lip*	*Tongue*	*Other Sites*
Etiology		Chronic irritation, leukoplakia	
Key words	1. Second most common site of oral cancer 2. Most common in males over 50 years 3. Carcinoma of upper lip uncommon 4. Best prognosis of all oral cancer	1. Most common site of oral cancer 2. Most common in males over 50 3. Most common site is lateral border 4. Anterior 2/3 tumors: 　a. more common 　b. better differentiated 　c. better prognosis than posterior 1/3 tumors 5. Extremely painful tumors (die from starvation)	1. Order of frequency: 　a. floor of mouth 　b. alveolar mucosa 　c. palate 　d. buccal mucosa 2. About 20% of oral malignancies are multicentric in origin

TUMORS OF THE SALIVARY GLANDS

General

1. Benign tumors of salivary glands much more common than malignant
2. Most common tumor of submaxillary gland is metastatic
3. Most common tumor of parotid gland is benign mixed
4. Of all primary parotid gland tumors 1/3 are malignant
5. Of all primary submaxillary gland tumors ½ are malignant
6. Salivary gland tumors of the lip more common in upper lip than in lower
7. Tumors of minor salivary glands can occur anywhere in oral cavity, but most common in hard palate

Benign Tumors of Salivary Glands

	Mixed Tumor (Pleomorphic Adenoma)	*Oxyphilic Adenoma (Oncocytoma)*	*Papillary Cystadenoma Lymphomatosum (Adenolymphoma; Warthin's Tumor)*
Clinical	Usually large	Usually small	Usually small
	Most common primary tumor of salivary glands	Very rare: under 1% of salivary gland tumors	Uncommon: about 5% of salivary gland tumors only 10% bilateral
	Usually seen in women about age 40	Usually unilateral	
	Usually unilateral		
Gross	Large bosselated mucoid tumors	Small solid tumor	Usually small with cystic spaces
Micro	MIXED epithelial and glandular elements with cartilage and mesenchymal cells May show calcification	Large polygonal cells with eosinophilic granules in cytoplasm (oncocysts)	Fluid-filled cystic spaces lined by *papillary projections* with lymphomatous-filled stromata projections lined by pseudostratified columnar epithelium with granular cytoplasm
EM		Cytoplasm of epithelial cells packed with mitochondria, some with vesicles containing glycogen	Cytoplasm of epithelial cells filled with mitochondria
Histogenesis	Both epithelial and mesodermal elements on tissue culture	Duct epithelium	Duct epithelium

(Continued on facing page)

Benign Tumors of Salivary Glands *(continued)*

	Mixed Tumor (Pleomorphic Adenoma)	Oxyphilic Adenoma (Oncocytoma)	Papillary Cystadenoma Lymphomatosum (Adenolymphoma) (Warthin's Tumor)
Special features	Malignant change: <5% Malignant mixed tumor: <5% of total mixed tumors NOT most common malignant tumor of salivary glands	Does not become malignant	Does not become malignant
	Recurrence common with incomplete excision: 5% 1st recurrence 25% 2nd recurrence	Rarely recurs	Rarely recurs
Key words	Damage to facial nerve with radical removal when parotid gland is involved		

Malignant Tumors of Salivary Glands: Some Peculiar Types*

Adenoid Cystic Carcinoma (Cylindromatous Adenocarcinoma)	Mucoepidermoid Carcinoma	Acinic Carcinoma
1. Well-differentiated tumor with cords and tubes (cylinders), formed mucin common 2. Early, wide metastases common 3. Looks benign in microscope, but behaves malignantly 4. Same micro as cylindromatous bronchial adenoma 5. Most common malignant tumor of submaxillary glands (AFIP)	1. Composed of 2 elements: a. mucin-producing cuboidal cells b. squamous cells with keratin formation 2. Malignant, metastasizes early and wide 3. Most common malignant tumor of parotid gland	1. Foamy clear cells with basophilic cytoplasm, arranged in acini 2. Resembles renal cell carcinoma 3. Clear cells NOT due to cytoplasmic fat or mucin: glycogen in small amounts in cells 4. Less malignant than others 5. 80% 5-year survival 6. Rare, about 1% of salivary gland tumors 7. More common in females 8. EM: cells contain multiple secretary granules

Almost all carcinomas of the salivary glands are variants of adenocarcinomas

Nonspecific Diseases of Salivary Glands

	Sjogren's Syndrome	Mikulicz's Disease	Uveoparotid Fever
Etiology	Unknown Autoimmune (?) disease	Unknown Variant of Sjogren's (?)	Now usually considered a form of sarcoidosis involving: uveal tract (choroid, iris, ciliary body), parotid glands, and frequently lacrimal gland.
Clinical	Full syndrome includes: 1. Keratoconjunctivitis sicca 2. Xerostomia 3. Recurrent parotid swelling 4. Rheumatoid arthritis 5. Most common in women over 40	Benign, systemic self-limiting syndrome No systemic symptoms Diffuse, chronic, asymptomatic enlargement of salivary or lacrimal glands	Usually with febrile course Most common in black females Usually with a triad of 1. Parotid enlargement 2. Uveitis 3. Facial paralysis (25%)
Pathology	Degeneration and atrophy of salivary glands (parotids) and lacrimal glands with chronic inflammatory cell infiltrate Micro: marked round cell, mostly lymphocyte and plasma cell infiltrate, with occasional germinal centers	Atrophy of acini with lymphoid cell infiltrates in glands Proliferation of epimyoepithelial islands of ductal Mikulicz cells in lumina of glands	Chronic noncaseating granulomatous nonspecific inflammation
Key words	1. Commonly show lack of phytohemagglutinin (PHA) transformation of lymphocytes 2. Hypergammaglobulinemia common 3. High incidence of lymphomas 4. FANA test positive in 40–75%	Do not confuse with Mikulicz's syndrome which is bilateral salivary gland enlargement due to any cause (usually lymphomas, sarcoidosis or TBC)	1. Now seen in about 10% of sarcoidosis cases 2. Spontaneous recovery common

12 Esophagus and Stomach

ESOPHAGUS

Diverticula

	Traction	Pulsion
Etiology	Tuberculous lymphadenitis	Unknown
Symptoms	Halitosis and dysphagia	Halitosis and dysphagia
Location	Lower 1/3 of esophagus or carina	Esophageal-pharyngeal junction, also just above cardia
Size	USUALLY small dimple	Often large
Special features	Less common Often painful Rarely large enough to collect food	More common MOST commonly collect food and cause symptoms

Carcinoma

	Squamous Cell Carcinoma	Adenocarcinoma
Relative incidence	90%	10%
Clinical	Common after age 50, males 5 : females 1, dysphagia, emaciation	
Location	Lower 1/3 MOST common (50%) Middle 1/3 (40%) Upper 1/3 (10%), usually with Plummer-Vinson syndrome	Lower 1/3 (90%)
Gross	1. Ulcerative 2. Polypoid 3. Diffuse infiltration	
Micro	Squamous cells with pearls and granulation tissue (desmoplasia)	Glands and stroma
Special features	1. Metastasizes or extends early because NO serosa present in esophagus 2. Does not usually metastasize widely; patients die of starvation or bronchopneumonia before cancer can spread widely 3. High correlation with cigarette smoking and alcohol use	

KEY FEATURES OF SPECIAL DISEASES AND SYNDROMES OF ESOPHAGUS

Plummer-Vinson Syndrome

1. Atrophic glossitis, dysphagia
2. Hypochromic microcytic anemia
3. Esophagitis (?) web
4. MOST common in middle-aged females
5. Esophagitis in upper 1/3 of esophagus
6. High incidence of carcinoma of upper 1/3 of esophagus
7. Syndrome treated with iron

Mallory-Weiss Syndrome

1. Esophageal lacerations at cardia
2. Associated with pernicious vomiting
3. Hematemesis also occurs
4. MOST common in alcoholics

Esophageal Varices

1. Associated with portal hypertension
2. Portal hypertension MOST commonly due to cirrhosis
3. Second most common cause of severe GI bleeding

Hiatal Hernia

	Sliding Hernia	*Rolling Hernia*
Etiology	Short esophagus, congenital or due to scarring	Cardia of stomach herniates alongside esophagus of normal length
Relative frequency	80%–90%	10%–20%
Clinical	10% have heartburn, regurgitation of gastric juice; 50% of patients with hiatal hernias on x-ray have no symptoms	
Pathology	Difficult to demonstrate at autopsy grossly, no diagnostic microscopic findings	
Notes	Higher incidence in patients with peptic ulcer disease Carcinoma is a rare complication	

Peptic Ulcers—Acute vs. Chronic

	Acute	*Chronic*
Etiology	1. Steroid therapy (Cushing's) 2. Uremia 3. Stress 4. Burns: Curling's ulcers	1. Unknown 2. Numerous factors (see Chronic Peptic Ulcers I)
Key words		
Number	Multiple	Usually single
Depth	Superficial	Deep
Location	Random	Lesser curvature and pylorus
Diameter	< 1 cm.	Usually about 2 cm.
Base color	Black, hemorrhagic	White, fibrous
Hemorrhages	Always	Frequent

Chronic Peptic Ulcers

	Stomach	*Duodenum*
Incidence	Males 4 : females 1; after menopause, males=females	
Etiology and pathogenic factors		
Cephalic phase	CNS, vagus, treated with tranquilizers, atropine, vagectomy	
Gastric phase	Gastrin, acid secretion, treated with antacids, mucosa coaters, gastrectomy	
Acid secretion	Normal or slightly up	High
Histamine response	Normal or slightly up	High
Parietal cell mass	Normal or low	2 × normal
Hormones, ACTH and corticosteroids	Increased incidence of ulcers, and increase in gastric and pepsin secretions	
Parathormone	Hyperparathyroidism; increased ulcers (calcium causes increased gastrin secretion)	
Sex hormones	Estrogens tend to protect from ulcers	
Blood type	Type O nonsecretors have 2 × normal incidence of ulcers (tend to be gastric)	
Emphysema	20% of emphysema patients have peptic ulcers; emphysema 3 times more common in ulcer patients than in general population	

(Continued on overleaf)

Chronic Peptic Ulcers *(continued)*

	Stomach	Duodenum
Drugs	Salicylates, reserpine, butazolidin, all cause increased incidence of ulcers	
Relative frequency	33%	66%
Location	1. Lesser curvature (64%) 2. Antrum (32%) 3. Greater curvature (1.9%)	1. Anterior wall, 1st portion 2. Posterior wall, 1st portion 3. 2nd portion
Size	SMALL, 75% < 3 cm. in diameter 50% < 2 cm. in diameter	
Anatomy	Round to oval, clean base, perpendicular wall, nonoverhanging, nonheaped-up margin	
Micro	Chronic inflammatory cell infiltrate, clean ACTIVE granulation tissue base	
Complications		
Order of occurrence	1. Pain 2. Hemorrhage 3. Perforation—5% of ulcers 4. Obstruction—very rare 5. Malignant transformation—less than 1%	1. Pain 2. Hemorrhage 3. Penetration into pancreas 4. Perforation: 5% of ulcers 5. Obstruction: more common than in stomach 6. Almost never malignant
Cause of death	(Overall less than 5% die of ulcers)	
	1. Perforation—65% of ulcer deaths 2. Massive hemorrhage: 25% of ulcer deaths 3. Obstruction, pylorus 4. Malignant transformation rare	1. Perforation—65% of ulcer deaths 2. Massive hemorrhage: 25% of ulcer deaths 3. Obstruction 4. Other

Ulcers of Stomach

	Benign	Malignant
Patient's age	USUALLY younger	USUALLY older
History	USUALLY long	USUALLY short
Gastric acidity	Normal to high	Often hypo- or achlorhydria
Blood group	Often Type O	Often Type A
Often associated conditions	Polycythemia Hyperparathyroidism Cushing's syndrome Rheumatoid arthritis with treatment	Pernicious anemia

Stomach Ulcer Morphology

	Benign	Malignant
Gross		
Size	USUALLY < 2 cm. diameter	USUALLY > 4 cm. diameter
Location	Lesser curvature, within 4–8 cm. of pylorus	1. Lesser curvature 2. Greater curvature
Base	Clean	Shaggy, dirty
Wall	Perpendicular	Often undermined
Margin	Flat	Heaped-up, overhanging
Micro	Inflammatory cells, granulation tissue	Cancer cells, granulation tissue (desmoplasia)

Common Benign Tumors of Stomach

Tumor	Relative Percentage of Benign Tumors of Stomach	Key Features
Adenoma	35%	1. USUALLY single but may be multiple 2. Polypoid cancer often develops from them
Leiomyoma	25%	1. Does not involve mucosa 2. MOST common benign tumor of GI tract 3. USUALLY small
Lipoma	5%	1. Does not involve mucosa 2. USUALLY small, without symptoms
Aberrant pancreas	3%	1. USUALLY around pylorus 2. More common in duodenal wall than in stomach

Carcinoma of the Stomach

	Ulcerative	Polypoid	Superficial Spreading (Linitis Plastica)
Clinical	MOST common in elderly males; associated with eating smoked fish in Iceland and Japan (nitrosamines ?) and with achlorhydria and pernicious anemia in U.S.A.		
Relative percentage	30%	25%	15%
Gross	Ulcer USUALLY > 4 cm. diameter Overhanging, heaped-up margin, dirty base	Large cauliflower masses, often from adenomas	Diffuse thickening of wall, "leather-bottle" stomach
Micro	Adenocarcinoma	Adenocarcinoma	Adenocarcinoma Tends to be signet-ring cell type
Prognosis	—————————— Less than 10% overall 5-year survival ——————————		
Special features	1. Virchow node: left supraclavicular area; common in stomach cancer but NOT pathognomonic, also occurs with lung, esophageal carcinomas and lymphomas 2. Krukenberg's tumor: bilateral ovarian tumor with signet-ring cells, originally from stomach; now, any GIT tumor with signet-ring cells involving ovaries		

OTHER MALIGNANT TUMORS OF STOMACH: KEY WORDS

Malignant Lymphoma

1. Second most common malignant tumor of stomach (3% of malignant stomach tumors —AFIP)
2. Usually discoid in distal ½ of stomach, but may have other patterns

Leiomyosarcoma

1. Third most common malignant tumor of stomach (1.7% of malignant stomach tumors— AFIP)
2. Probably arises from leiomyomas, which are quite common

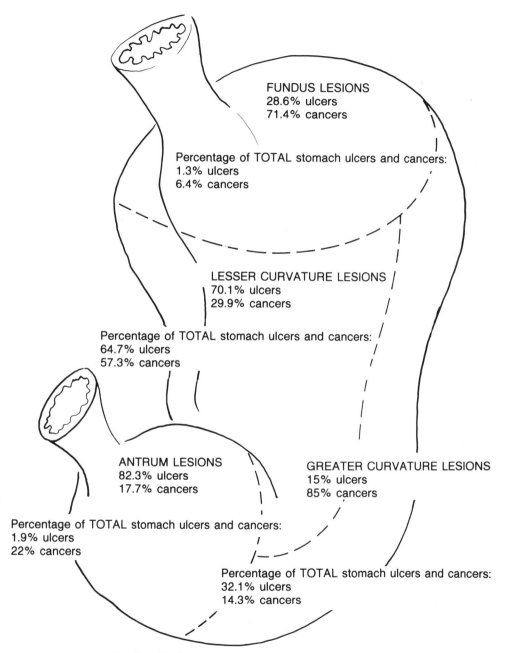

FUNDUS LESIONS
28.6% ulcers
71.4% cancers

Percentage of TOTAL stomach ulcers and cancers:
1.3% ulcers
6.4% cancers

LESSER CURVATURE LESIONS
70.1% ulcers
29.9% cancers

Percentage of TOTAL stomach ulcers and cancers:
64.7% ulcers
57.3% cancers

ANTRUM LESIONS
82.3% ulcers
17.7% cancers

GREATER CURVATURE LESIONS
15% ulcers
85% cancers

Percentage of TOTAL stomach ulcers and cancers:
1.9% ulcers
22% cancers

Percentage of TOTAL stomach ulcers and cancers:
32.1% ulcers
14.3% cancers

Fig. 12–1. Distribution of benign and malignant gastric lesions.

Principal Bleeding Lesions in 135 Deaths from Gastrointestinal Hemorrhage

Lesion	Cases	Percent
Peptic ulcerations	50	37.0
Esophagus	7	
Stomach	10	
Acute ulcers and erosions	2	
Subacute and chronic ulcers	8	
Duodenum	31	
Esophagus, stomach and duodenum	1	
Stomach and duodenum (chronic)	1	
Esophageal varices	43	31.9
Neoplastic ulcerations	20	14.8
Stomach	10	
Pancreas	6	
Esophagus	2	
Duodenum	2	
Blood dyscrasia	11	8.1
Biliary tract (postoperative)	4	3.0
No lesion found	4	3.0
Miscellaneous	3	2.2
Infarction of stomach and intestines	1	
Aneurysm of hepatic artery	1	
Dissecting hematoma	1	
Total	135	100.0

PRINCIPAL CAUSES OF SIGNIFICANT NONFATAL GASTROINTESTINAL HEMORRHAGE

Noncirrhotic Patients

Chronic peptic ulcer 35%
  a. duodenum (25%)
  b. stomach   (10%)
  c. total   (35%)
Esophageal varices 18%
Erosive gastritis 14%
Undetermined site 10%
All other causes (each < 5%) 23%

Cirrhotic Patients

Chronic peptic ulcer 20%
  a. duodenum (14%)
  b. stomach   (6%)
  c. total   (20%)
Esophageal and gastric varices 53%
Gastritis 22%
No cause found 5%

13 Small Intestine

Malabsorption Syndromes

Nontropical Sprue (Gluten Enteropathy; Celiac Disease)	Tropical Sprue	Intestinal Lipodystrophy (Whipple's Disease)

Etiology

1. Gluten (wheat) toxicity hypersensitivity
2. Lack of peptidase to split gliadin peptides
3. Nontropical sprue (adults)
4. Celiac disease (children)
	1. Occurs in tropics
	2. Folic acid deficiency (?)
	3. Microbiological etiology (?)
	4. Occurs in epidemics
		1. Unknown etiology
		   a. microbiological (?), bacilliform bodies
		   b. lysosomal (?), genetic (?)
		2. Males 8 : females 1
		3. Develop marked wasting

Clinical

—————— Weight loss, bulky, foul-smelling stools, steatorrhea, diarrhea ——————

Gross

Unremarkable, to slightly flattened Kerckring valves and loss of velvety appearance of mucosa	1. Thickened wall of small intestine, swollen mesentery 2. Mucosa: shaggy, "bearskin rug"

Micro

Atrophy and blunting of villi, chronic inflammatory cell infiltrate in lamina propria of jejunum	1. Clubbed, blunted villi 2. Foamy, (glycoprotein) PAS-positive macrophages in lamina propria and lymphatics 3. Lipogranulomas with ruptured lacteals

EM

1. Shortened, distorted microvilli 2. Abnormal mitochondria 3. Disaggregation of ribosomes 4. Organelles into terminal web area	Bacilliform bodies free or in vesicles, secondary lysosomes (telolysosomes ?) "Sickle-form" (?) bodies in histiocytes

74

(Continued on facing page)

Malabsorption Syndromes *(continued)*

Nontropical Sprue (Gluten Enteropathy) (Celiac Disease)	Tropical Sprue	Intestinal Lipodystrophy (Whipple's Disease)

Special Features

Nontropical Sprue (Gluten Enteropathy) (Celiac Disease)	Tropical Sprue	Intestinal Lipodystrophy (Whipple's Disease)
1. Often treated with gluten-free diet 2. Some have increased IgA levels 3. Some have IgA on BM after gluten challenge	1. Gluten-free diet does not treat 2. Sometimes treated with antibiotics 3. Some respond to B_{12} and folic acid	1. Can often diagnose with rectal biopsy: PAS-positive histiocytes 2. Also may have arthritis and other systemic symptoms 3. Bacilliform bodies disappear and many patients are well in 6 months when Rxed with tetracyclines

Regional Enteritis vs. Ulcerative Colitis

	Regional (Ileitis) Enteritis (Crohn's Disease)	Ulcerative Colitis
Etiology	Unknown, emotional (?) hypersensitivity (?)	Unknown—emotional (?), auto-immune
Associated systemic conditions	None known, NOT sarcoid	Psoriasis—5% Rheumatoid arthritis-like syndrome 20% Cirrhosis—5%–10%
Incidence	Age 20–40 NOT common	Age 20–40 Not uncommon
Sex	Males = females	Males = females
Symptoms	Intermittent pain, melena, constipation	Intermittent pain, diarrhea; mucus, blood in stool
Gross		
Location	Terminal ileum most common, 80% of cases Colon involved in 40% of cases (called segmental colitis there) Skip lesions	Colon, 75% of cases Rectosigmoid most common Ileum: 15%–20% of cases NO skip lesions
Appearance	Wall very thick "Rubber hose" "Eel in rigor mortis" X-ray string sign All layers involved, may extend to mesentery	Wall moderately thickened Most severe in mucosa and submucosa Ulcers over teniae coli Pseudopolyps (normal edematous mucosa) between ulcers
Micro	Sarcoid-like (noncaseating) granulomas and chronic inflammation in over 80%	Nonspecific Chronic inflammation NO granulomas Paneth cells commonly abundant
Complications	1. Obstruction 2. Perforation, fistula 3. NO malignancy 4. Clubbing of fingers rare	1. Perforation, fistula, peritonitis 2. Malignancy about 10% of cases 3. Clubbing of fingers rare to uncommon
Notes	1. Can have both conditions in same patient 2. Regional enteritis also known as transmural colitis	

Diverticula of Intestines

	Small Intestine	*Large Intestine*
Etiology	Congenital	(?) Congenital, increased intraluminal pressure and muscle atrophy
Incidence	Duodenum most common, less than 1% of population Jejunum and ileum, rarer	5% of population over age 50, 25% over age 65
Number	Single to a few	Always multiple
Size	USUALLY large	USUALLY small
Location	Mesenteric border	Along edge of teniae coli Mostly in sigmoid and rectum
Special features	USUALLY asymptomatic May have blind-loop syndrome with macrocytic anemia	1. USUALLY have some pain USUALLY intermittent symptoms 2. Tend to get plugged up and inflamed, may perforate 3. Complications: a. perforation: fistulas, peritonitis b. obstruction c. hemorrhage

Meckel's Diverticulum

What is it?	Remnant of omphalomesenteric duct
Location	TWO feet from ileocecal valve on ANTImesenteric border of ileum
Size	TWO inches long
Diameter	TWO centimeters
Incidence	TWO % of population
Other features	1. 50% have heterotopic gastric mucosa 2. Less than 50% have heterotopic pancreas 3. May have ulcers at margin of diverticulum

Special Small Bowel Syndromes

Carcinoid Syndrome	Zollinger-Ellison Syndrome	Enteric Coated Potassium Syndrome

Etiology and pathogenesis

Carcinoid Syndrome	Zollinger-Ellison Syndrome	Enteric Coated Potassium Syndrome
Tumor arising from Kulchitsky (argentaffin) cells	Noninsulin, (?) gastrin-secreting tumor of pancreas	Enteric coated KCl tablets in patients on thiazide diuretics

Signs and symptoms

Flushing, blushing, diarrhea, right-sided heart failure, murmurs	Chronic peptic ulcers USUALLY in duodenum, may have diarrhea	Diarrhea, electrolyte imbalance

Gross

Yellow, firm, small, MOST common in appendix, 60% (Almost never metastasize) Extra-appendiceal: 1. Small bowel (2/3) 2. Stomach 3. Large bowel	90%: firm, gray tumor up to 2 cm. diameter in pancreas 10%: no gross lesions	1. Lesion mostly in jejunum, but may be in ileum 2. Early: focal hemorrhage and edema 3. Later: SEGMENTAL scarring and fibrosis

Micro

Small clusters of ovoid cells in nests and cords	Nests of usually BENIGN-LOOKING islet cells	Congestion, hemorrhage— granulomas

Special Features

1. Need liver metastases to get syndrome 2. 40% of extra-appendiceal carcinoids metastasize 3. HIAA in urine to diagnose	1. 60% of tumors are malignant, 2/3 of these metastasize 2. 30% adenomas 3. 10% hyperplasia of islets 4. 25% of ulcers located in atypical locations (e.g., jejunum) 5. May have adenomas of other endocrine organs 6. May be part of MEA I (See Chap. 19)	1. May confuse with regional enteritis 2. Enteric coated potassium tablets are being removed from market in U.S.A.

14 Large Intestine

Carcinoma of Large Bowel

Incidence	Males and females equally affected Overall MOST common carcinoma; excluding skin MOST common after age 50	
Predisposing conditions	1. Villous adenoma 2. Ulcerative colitis 3. Adenomatous (?) polyps 4. Familial polyposis	
Location	Approximately 2/3 within reach of sigmoidoscope	
	Right-sided Lesion	*Left-sided Lesion*
Symptoms	1. Late 2. Weakness, malaise, anemia 3. Guaiac-positive stools	1. Earlier 2. Obstipation 3. Constipation 4. Pencil stools
Gross	Polypoid, fungating; with obstruction late	Napkin-ring lesion, obstruction early
Micro	Adenocarcinoma, often with mucin	Adenocarcinoma, often with mucin
Diagnoses	*Dukes' (1937) Classification*	*5-Year Survival*
	Confined to bowel wall	85%
	Serosa but NOT beyond	70%
	Serosa and beyond	25%
Survival	Overall 5 years	25%–40%
	With over 6 nodes involved	10%
	With over 15 nodes involved	0%
Notes	1. Carcinoembryonic antigen (CEA) positive in about 1/3 of cases without metastasis and up to 95% of cases with metastasis 2. CEA not specific; also positive in many other tumors and diseases including heavy cigarette smoking 3. CEA most useful as a screening test, and if positive, is useful as a marker test for tumor recurrence after Rx	

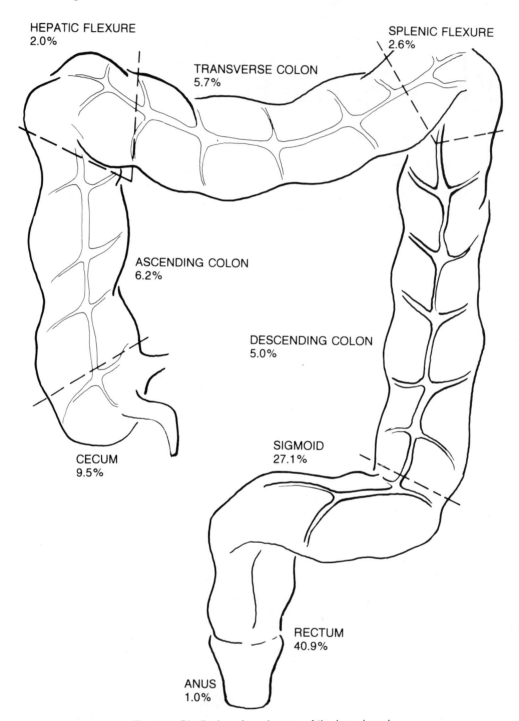

HEPATIC FLEXURE
2.0%

SPLENIC FLEXURE
2.6%

TRANSVERSE COLON
5.7%

ASCENDING COLON
6.2%

DESCENDING COLON
5.0%

CECUM
9.5%

SIGMOID
27.1%

RECTUM
40.9%

ANUS
1.0%

Fig. 14–1. Distribution of carcinomas of the large bowel.

Polyps I

	Adenomatous Polyp	*Villous Adenoma*
Incidence	10% of population over age 50	Unknown, < 0.5% of persons over age 50
Sex	No sex preponderance	No sex preponderance
Symptoms	Usually none, or diarrhea, bloody stool	Usually none, or bloody stool and diarrhea
Gross		
Number	Often more than one	USUALLY singular
Location	More uniform distribution in large bowel than villous adenoma	75% in rectosigmoid
Appearance	Have stalk (PEDUNCULATED)	No stalk (SESSILE)
Micro	Most are < 3 cm. in diameter Adenomatous hyperplastic glands	Most are 5 cm. in diameter Long fronds with hyperplastic or anaplastic epithelial cells extending from mucosa to lumen
Complications	1. Obstruction 2. May be leading edge of intussusception 3. Up to 5% become malignant 4. Rectal bleeding	1. Considered a PREMALIGNANT condition, over 70% become or show focal malignancy 2. Electrolyte imbalance, secrete potassium and absorb chloride, hypokalemic alkalosis

Polyps II

	Familial Polyposis	*Peutz-Jeghers Syndrome*	*Other Polypoid Syndromes*
Incidence and syndrome	Rare, autosomal dominant, age 20 to 40	Rare, autosomal dominant, polyps of small and large bowel with melanin pigmentation of buccal mucosa and lips	1. Gardner's syndrome (rare) a. polyps of colon b. associated neoplasm elsewhere c. autosomal dominant 2. Turcot syndrome (rare) a. polyps of colon b. brain tumors c. autosomal recessive

(Continued on overleaf)

Polyps II *(continued)*

	Familial Polyposis	Peutz-Jeghers Syndrome	Other Polyploid Syndromes
Gross			
Number and location	Multiple from cecum to anus, may involve small intestine or stomach	Polyps, multiple	All produce multiple adenomatous polyps
Size	Small, 1–2 cm. pedunculated, adenomatous polyps	Pedunculated, small, of entire GI tract including small intestine	Variable, small
Micro	Hyperplastic glands, stroma	Identical to adenomatous polyps	Identical to adenomatous polyps
Special features	70%–100% develop adenocarcinoma if not resected	RARELY develop cancer	Polyps may become malignant

Polyps III

	Juvenile (Retention) Polyps	Other Benign Polyps
Incidence	In children, usually under age 5 (In adults called retention polyps)	All are uncommon
Symptoms	Rectal bleeding in 80% (a cause of currant-jelly stools in children) Protruding mass in 25%	Rectal bleeding or diarrhea 1. Lipomatous polyp 2. Leiomyomatous polyp 3. Lymphomatous polyp
Gross		
Location	MOST common in rectosigmoid	Anywhere in GI tract
Size	1–3 cm. in diameter, usually singular, may or may not have stalk	All usually 1–4 cm. in diameter and singular USUALLY do not involve mucosa
Micro	Composed of GRANULATION TISSUE, often with cystic dilated glands	1. Mature fat tissue 2. Whorled smooth muscle 3. Hyperplastic lymphoid tissue
Special features	1. Often seen as leading edge for intussusception 2. NEVER become malignant	1. Very low malignant potential 2. May be leading edge for intussusception 3. May cause rectal bleeding

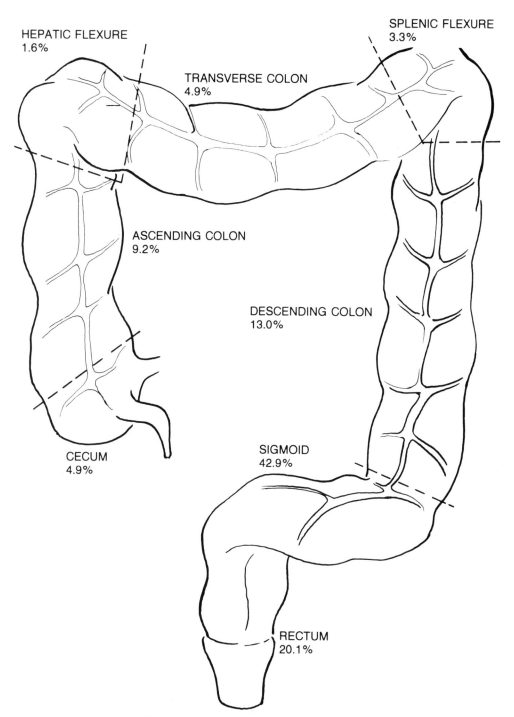

HEPATIC FLEXURE
1.6%

SPLENIC FLEXURE
3.3%

TRANSVERSE COLON
4.9%

ASCENDING COLON
9.2%

DESCENDING COLON
13.0%

CECUM
4.9%

SIGMOID
42.9%

RECTUM
20.1%

Fig. 14–2. Distribution of polyps of the large bowel.

Dysentery

	Bacillary	Amebic
Type of lesion	Suppurative	Necrotic
Symptoms	Diarrhea, bloody, mucous stools	Diarrhea, bloody, mucous stools
Organism	*Shigella dysenteriae*	*Entamoeba histolytica* up to 4 nuclei
Ulcer		

Depth
  Wall margin
  Wall itself
  Base
	USUALLY shallow, long axis
	Sharp
	NOT undermined
	Shaggy
		USUALLY deep
		Ragged
		Undermined, flask-shaped
		Necrotic

Micro	Polys and acute inflammation	Mononuclear cells and organisms, erythrophagocytosis
Mucosa between ulcers	Inflamed with fibrinosuppurative membrane (pseudomembrane)	Normal
Cytology of stools	Polymorphonuclears	Mononuclears + Charcot-Leyden crystals
Liver abscess	Almost never, because shigella do not get into blood	Common (about 40% of cases)
Complications	Dehydration and electrolyte imbalance in either Perforation may occur with either	

Mechanical Intestinal Obstruction

Most Common Causes	Percentage of Mechanical Obstruction
1. Adhesions	50%
2. Hernias	25%
3. Intussusception	10%
4. Volvulus	4%

HIRSCHSPRUNG'S DISEASE (CONGENITAL MEGACOLON): KEY WORDS

1. Dilated colon PROXIMAL to aganglionic colon (loss of Meissner's and Auerbach's plexuses)
2. MOST common in rectosigmoid area, also occurs in ureters
3. Can usually diagnose by rectal biopsy

15 Liver–Except Cirrhosis

Hepatitis I

	Hepatitis A	Hepatitis B
Synonyms	Infectious hepatitis (IH) MS-1 HA Ab-Positive hepatitis	Serum hepatitis (SH) MS-2 HBs Ag-Positive hepatitis
Etiology	Enterovirus with RNA, 27 nm. diameter	DNA virus (Dane particle) 42 nm., composed of core antigen (HBc Ag) and surface antigen (HBs Ag)
Incubation period (from exposure to SGOT 2 times normal)	15–40 days	50–160 days (much longer if orally acquired)
Age group	Usually children and young adults	All age groups
Jaundice	———————— Rare in children, more common in adults ————————	
HAA (HBs Ag) (Australia antigen in blood)	No	25%–90% of cases
Virus in feces	Yes	No
Virus in blood	Present during late incubation period and early acute phase	HBs Ag present during late incubation period and early acute phase, usually absent before bilirubin rises, occasionally persists for months or years ("carriers"), HBc Ag present during acute infection
Immunity Homologous Heterologous	Present None	Unknown None
Gamma globulin prophylaxis	Excellent	Generally poor, but high anti-HBs titer serum seems to protect

Hepatitis I *(continued)*

	Hepatitis A	Hepatitis B
Pathology	Cannot distinguish between the two on morphologic grounds, but SH usually more severe than IH	
Gross	Liver is soft, nearly normal in size, with yellow-red mottling	
Micro and EM	1. Diffuse lobular disorganization 2. Balloon degeneration, dilated cisternae of ER and mitochondria, ? virus-like particles in cytoplasm and nucleus 3. Focal hepatic necrosis and inflammation 4. Eosinophilic (acidophilic) bodies in Kupffer cells resemble Councilman bodies 5. Portal mononuclear cell infiltrates 6. Absence of stainable neutral fat	
Key words	All will regenerate if reticular framework is intact	
Prognosis	1. Death under 1% 2. 95% have complete recovery	1. Death up to 12% 2. About 85% have complete recovery
Complications	Acute yellow atrophy (fulminant hepatitis) Post-hepatitic or postnecrotic cirrhosis Cholangitis—interhepatic cholestasis (cholestatic hepatitis), micro same as allergic type drug cholestasis Chronic progressive or persistent hepatitis (see below)	

VIRAL HEPATITIS NOTES

1. 0.5% of USA population carries HB_sAg
2. 20% of young urban adult serum contains anti-HB_s
3. There are several subtypes of HB_sAg (e.g., a,d,w,y)
4. In spite of universal HB_sAg detection, the incidence of posttransfusion hepatitis is high (e.g., 20% of cardiac bypass patients get elevated SGOT 3 months post-surgery and 20% of these get icteric disease. 80% of post-transfusion hepatitis patients have no evidence of hepatitis A or B antigens

Is there a Hepatitis C? Conrad, M.E. and Knodell, R.G.: (*JAMA, 233*:1277–1278, 1975)

Hepatitis C (non-A, non-B Hepatitis)

Evidence for its existence
1. Above evidence that 80% of posttransfusion hepatitis is non-A, non-B
2. Epstein-Barr virus: most patients with infectious mononucleosis get at least a chemical "hepatitis" with elevations of one or more of the following: SGOT, bilirubin and alkaline phosphatase. Some develop full-blown "hepatitis" syndrome
3. Cytomegalic virus has been implicated in some "hepatitis" cases

THE VARIANTS OF HEPATITIS

General

Hepatologists have developed a bewildering array of names and subclassifications for the *persistent, recurrent,* and *chronic* stages of viral hepatitis. The currently known variants with key features are shown in the following tables. Besides those listed in table form, the following are used for variants of hepatitis:

Chronic Submassive Hepatitis

A severe ongoing hepatitis; less severe than fulminant hepatitis, goes to pre-cirrhosis in most cases.

Cholangiolytic or Cholestatic Hepatitis

1. Variant of hepatitis with severe verdinic jaundice, pruritus, bilirubin over 15 mg% and bile acid retention
2. Biopsy often shows more marked bile duct involvement than classic cases of hepatitis
3. It is supposed that this type of hepatitis goes to a biliary cirrhosis more frequently than the classic type of hepatitis

Relapsing Hepatitis

1. Hepatitis patients who become biochemically normal, then develop abnormal liver function tests (LFT) and/or symptoms
2. Said to occur in 10–15% of acute hepatitis patients within 1st year
3. Difficult to differentiate from chronic hepatitis

Anicteric Hepatitis

1. Hepatitis A, B or (? C) without clinical jaundice
2. A self-limited disease in most cases

Hepatitis—Persistent Variants

	Chronic ($HB_S Ag$) Carriers	Chronic Persistent Hepatitis (Acute Prolonged Hepatitis)
Approximate frequency	0.02–0.34% of general population (blood bank data) About 2–5% of viral hepatitis $HB_S Ag$ positive will become carriers	Under 5% of acute viral hepatitis cases
Proposed pathogenesis	Inadequate $HB_S Ag$ responses (in cytoplasm "ground glass hepatocytes"?) with normal $HB_C Ag$ responses in nucleus ? abnormal T cell function	Impaired antibody (B and T cell) response $HB_C Ag$ persists in nucleus with minimal tissue injury
Morphologic pattern	Usually normal May show portal mononuclear cells. Rarely shows focal intralobular necrosis	Portal mononuclear (lymphocyte, plasma cell and monocyte) infiltration with occasional focal hepatocyte necrosis
Key features	1. Most show normal LFT 2. Some may show LFT abnormalities	1. Show elevated SGOT, SGPT. $HB_S Ag$ may be detected 2. Higher incidence of lymphomas, leukemias, and uremia 3. Difficult or impossible to differentiate from relapsing hepatitis
Prognosis	Usually excellent	Good–excellent
Viral type	B only, by definition	B and, possibly, A

Hepatitis—Progressive Variants

	Chronic Active Hepatitis Chronic Agressive Hepatitis	Fulminant Hepatitis, Massive Hepatic Necrosis, Acute Yellow Atrophy
Approximate frequency	About 5% of acute hepatitis B patients	Under 5% of acute hepatitis cases Frequently associated with hepatitis B and illicit drug injection
Proposed pathogenesis	Inadequate antibody response to both HB_S and $HB_C Ag$ with persistence of both in hepatocytes with cell injury Cytotoxic lymphocytes cause injury	? Excessive antibody response causing widespread cellular destruction
Morphologic patterns	"Piecemeal necrosis", bridging, periportal or central necrosis and fibrosis and multilobular necrosis and fibrosis, mononuclears in portal area	Bridging, multilobular and submassive necrosis. Grossly yellow-red mottled liver with wrinkled capsule
Key features	1. All have abnormal LFT 2. Over 50% of patients with portal bridging necrosis progress to post-necrotic cirrhosis 3. Require continued steroid Rx to control 4. High incidence of HLA-1 and HLA-8 5. About 2/3 have AMA antibodies 6. 85% have anti-smooth-muscle antibodies 7. Most are $HB_S Ag$ positive	1. Clinically: nausea, vomiting, deepening jaundice and obtundency are seen 2. Massively abnormal LFT, hypoalbuminemia, high blood NH_3 are seen 3. Those that survive acute attack frequently have postnecrotic cirrhosis 4. There is no effective therapy
Prognosis	Fair-poor, over 50% go to postnecrotic cirrhosis	Poor, 80% mortality
Virus type	B	B and, uncommonly, A

Lupoid Hepatitis

1. Probably identical to, or indistinguishable from, chronic active hepatitis
2. Typical patient is female, with positive LE prep and FANA test
3. Morphologically similar to chronic active hepatitis

Neonatal (Giant Cell) Hepatitis

1. Seen ONLY in newborn infants
2. Liver large
3. Parenchymal cells replaced by multinucleate giant cells, dense bodies (iron-bilirubin complex) present in cytoplasm of giant cells with EM
4. Marked bile stasis with loss of bile canaliculi
5. Lobular disarray
6. Probably NOT due to a virus
7. Some recover
8. Must distinguish from congenital biliary atresia (dense bodies help)

LIVER TUMORS

Benign
Cavernous hemangioma most common primary benign tumor of liver

Malignant
Metastatic most common malignant tumor in liver

PRIMARY TUMORS

Hepatoma (Hepatocellular)
1. Most common type, rare in U.S.A.
2. 50%–80% associated with cirrhosis in U.S.A.
3. Arises in postnecrotic cirrhosis more often than in Laennec's cirrhosis
4. Usually multicentric in origin
5. 66% of cases have fetoprotein associated
6. Thorotrast, butter-yellow, aflatoxins, *Clonorchis sinensis* and schistosomes are known causes
7. Micro: hyperplastic liver cells

Cholangiocarcinoma
1. Least common carcinoma of liver
2. Less frequently associated with cirrhosis than hepatocellular carcinoma
3. Micro: usually an adenocarcinoma
4. Often have mixed hepatoma—cholangiocarcinoma

Angiosarcoma of Liver
1. A very rare lesion in in the general population
2. Common in industrial exposure to vinyl chloride monomer
3. See Chap. 10 for more details

Drug and Chemical Injury of Liver

	"Predictable" Drug Reactions		*"Idiosyncratic" Drug Reactions*	
	Chemical Necrosis	*Pure Cholestasis*	*Mixed Cholestasis—Hepatocellular Necrosis (Allergic Drug Injury)*	*Toxic Hepatitis*
Classically caused by	*Centrilobular Necrosis* 1. Carbon tetrachloride 2. Chloroform 3. Alcohol 4. TNT *Peripheral Lobular Necrosis* 1. Phosphorus 2. Eclampsia *Midzonal Necrosis* Yellow fever	1. Steroids 2. Methyltestos-terone 3. Chlorpromazine 4. The Pill ? predictable	1. Chlorpromazine 2. Antibiotics, including sulfas and tetracycline (fine droplet accumulation with tetracycline) 3. Antidiabetic compounds 4. Most common type of drug reaction	1. Isoniazid, PAS 2. MAO inhibitors 3. Halothane 4. Tetracycline in 3rd trimester of pregnancy 5. Dilantin
Pathology	1. Areas of fatty change and frank necrosis of liver cells with inflammation 2. Distribution often characteristic of etiologic agent	1. Canalicular plugging 2. Rarely some hepatic cell degeneration 3. Blunted or absent microvilli of hepatocytes	1. Severe centricanalicular cholestasis 2. Marked triaditis: neutrophils, eosinophils and mononuclear cells 3. Single-cell hepatic necrosis 4. Preservation of lobular architecture 5. Anisocytosis of hepatic cells 6. Atypical ductular proliferation in portal spaces	1. Morphologically indistinguishable from viral hepatitis 2. EM: proliferated SER and Golgi (see Hepatitis I) 3. Massive necrosis (see hepatitis, above)

Miscellaneous Conditions of the Liver: Key Words

Budd-Chiari Syndrome (Rare)	*Cholangitis (Ascending)*	*Peliosis Hepatitis (Rare)*

1. Thrombotic hepatic vein occlusion
2. Most commonly due to
  a. endophlebitis (2/3)
  b. polycythemia vera
  c. renal cell carcinoma
  d. cirrhosis of liver
3. Symptoms
  a. rapid onset of ascites (NO ascites in portal vein thrombosis)
  b. enlarging liver and abdominal pain
	1. Most common organism *E. coli*
	2. Most commonly due to ascending inflammation of bile duct due to obstruction by stone or cancer
		1. Multiple small blood-filled spaces throughout liver
		2. Most often seen with prolonged steroid therapy
		3. Also seen in patients dying of TBC

Cholestasis

	Extrahepatic	Intrahepatic
General	More common Most commonly due to (a) stones, (b) cancer	Less common Usually associated with viral hepatitis
Alkaline phosphatase	4+	4+
Pathology	Central canalicular intrahepatic cholestasis	Central canalicular intrahepatic cholestasis
Diagnostic	1. Inspissated bile in interlobular ducts 2. Bile lakes 3. Bile necrosis (infarcts)	Same as acute viral hepatitis, often difficult to distinguish from drug-induced cholestasis
Suggestive	1. Concentric fibrosis around interlobular ducts 2. Feathery degeneration of hepatic cells 3. Foam cells, hepatic and Kupffer 4. Typical ductular proliferation 5. Acute portal inflammation	
Electron microscope	Dilated, plugged bile canaliculi with atrophy of microvilli	1. Myelin sheathlike SER 2. Lysosomes (autophagic) 3. Giant MITOCHONDRIA 4. Swelling and edema of microvilli

Notes 1. Liver biopsy cannot distinguish 25% of the time between extrahepatic and intrahepatic cholestasis
   2. In advanced cases, the AMA test is positive in a large number of *intra*hepatic cases and negative in *extra*hepatic cases.

16 Liver–Cirrhosis

Fatty Nutritional (Alcoholic) Laennec's Cirrhosis

	Early *Alcoholic Hepatitis*	*Middle* *Classic*	*Late* *END STAGE LIVER*
Etiology	——————————— Prolonged heavy drinking ———————————		
Pathogenesis	Direct damage to liver by alcohol (?), average duration of drinking about 5 years Excess alcohol; lack of lipotrophic factors (methionine, choline, selenium, vitamin E)		
Clinical	Most common type of cirrhosis in U.S.A., rare in Scotland More common in men than women For signs and symptoms, see page 96		
Pathology			
Gross	Liver large	Normal size	Atrophic liver
Weight	Large–to 6000 g.	1800–2000 g.	1200 g.
Color	Yellow	Yellow-brown, umber	Nearly normal
External surface	Smooth, "greasy"	Uniform small nodules, fine scars, hobnail, 0.2–0.3 cm.	Hobnail, uniform, large nodules, 0.5–1.0 cm., fine scars
Cut surface	Smooth, soft, NO nodules	Firm, uniform, small nodules, 0.2–0.3 cm.	Very firm, uniform, nodules, 0.5–1.0 cm.

(Continued on facing page)

Fatty Nutritional (Alcoholic) Laennec's Cirrhosis *(continued)*

	Early Alcoholic Hepatitis	Middle Classic	Late END STAGE LIVER
Micro			
Fat	4+	2+	+−
Fibrous tissue	+−	2+ (stellate)	4+
Intact lobules	4+	1+	+−
Pseudolobulation	0	3+	3−4+
Bile duct proliferation	0	1+	1+
Hemosiderin	0	1+	1+
Bile stasis	1+	1+	1+
Central vein intact	3+	1+	+−
Portal neutrophils	4+	2+	+−
Focal hepatic cell necrosis	3+	2+	1+
Alcoholic hyaline (Mallory bodies)	4+	2+	+−
	Their presence and number may imply poorer prognosis		

Special features	1. Low incidence of hepatoma with alcoholic cirrhosis
	2. Nodules of regeneration in all types of cirrhosis show liver plates two cells thick
	3. ¼ to 1/3 of patients with alcoholic cirrhosis show no symptoms of cirrhosis
	4. Mortality after onset of symptoms:
	   a. within 1 year 50%
	   b. within 3 years 75%

EM	Bizarre large mitochondria with stacking of cristae

Posthepatitic vs. Postnecrotic Cirrhosis

	Posthepatitic	Postnecrotic
Etiology and pathogenesis	1. Most cases etiology unknown 2. (?) Due to mild attacks of hepatitis; viral, bacterial 3. Can produce experimentally by multiple light exposures to hepatotoxins	1. After severe attack of viral or acute yellow atrophy 2. Can produce experimentally by massive exposure to hepatotoxins
Clinical	Incidence controversial 1. Common, over ½ of cirrhosis cases in one series 2. Rare, in most series	Symptoms usually develop soon after attack of hepatitis
Pathology		
Gross	Normal early, to 1000 g. late	Normal early, to 600 g. late
Color	Reddish brown, with fine scars	Gray-brown with coarse scars
External surface	Hobnail *trabecular* scars	*Irregular,* broad scarring

(Continued on overleaf)

Posthepatic vs. Postnecrotic Cirrhosis *(continued)*

	Posthepatitic	*Postnecrotic*
Cut surface	Nodules uniform, coarse 0.5–1.0 cm., every portal area is involved	Nodules irregular, 0.3–5.0 cm.
Micro		
Fat	0	+−
Fibrous tissue	3+ (trabecular scars)	4+ (broad scars)
Intact lobules	4+	1+ (irregular)
Pseudolobulations	0	2+
Bile duct Proliferation	1+	3+
Hemosiderin	0	+−
Central vein intact	4+	+− (some areas)
Portal inflammation	4+ (lymphocytes)	1+
Focal hepatic cell necrosis	1+	4+
Mallory bodies	No	No
Special features	1. Scars mainly follow normal outlines of liver and rarely cut across liver lobules 2. 5% to 6% of normal population have it to some degree	1. Broad areas of scarring due to collapsed lobules 2. Hepatomas most commonly occur with this type of cirrhosis 3. *Most* common type of cirrhosis in England

Biliary Cirrhosis

	Primary (Hanot's) Cirrhosis	*Secondary Biliary Obstructive Cirrhosis*
Etiology and pathology	1. Unknown 2. Drugs, methyltestosterone, chlorpromazine 3. NO biliary tract obstruction 4. Autoimmune, can detect gamma globulin with fluorescent antibodies	1. Secondary to EXTRAhepatic bile duct obstruction most commonly due to: a. stone in common bile duct b. tumor at head of pancreas, ampulla of Vater
Clinical	——————————— Verdinic jaundice ——————————— ————— Pruritus a very common sequela due to bile salts ————— Most common in middle-aged females	Difficult to differentiate from primary biliary cirrhosis (symptoms and signs often identical)
Pathology		
Gross	Enlarged	Usually normal, but may be enlarged
Color	Dark green	Dark green

(Continued on facing page)

Biliary Cirrhosis *(continued)*

	Primary (Hanot's) Cirrhosis	*Secondary Biliary Obstructive Cirrhosis*
External surface	Tough, granular	Tough, granular
Cut surface	Granular, firm	Fine nodules, granular (?)
Micro		
Fat	1+	1+
Fibrous tissue	2+ (around triads and is monolobular)	3+ (same as in portal cirrhosis—alcoholic)
Intact lobules	4+	2+
Pseudolobulation	1+	2+
Bile duct proliferation	2+ (loss of finest bile duct radicals)	4+
Hemosiderin	1+	1+
Central vein intact	3+	2+
Portal inflammation	4+ (plasma cells)	3+ (polys or mononuclear cells)
Local hepatic cell necrosis	3+ (around triads)	1+
Mallory bodies	No	No
Bile lakes	2+	4+ (with bile infarcts and polys)
Special features	1. Can often differentiate from secondary by serum immunofluorescence tests 2. With high plasma lipids, can get xanthomas (xanthomatous biliary cirrhosis)	1. MUCH more common than intrahepatic type 2. Marked jaundice but NO ascites
Serum alkaline phosphatase level	4+	4+
Antimitochondrial and smooth muscle antibody	3+ (to 90%)	Negative

Pigmentary, Cardiac-Congestive and Hepar Lobatum Cirrhosis

	Pigmentary	*Cardiac-Congestive*	*Hepar Lobatum*
Etiology and pathogenesis	Part of hemochromatosis Men 9 : 1	1. Very, very rare 2. Due to severe long-standing CPC 3. Some doubt its existence	Part of tertiary syphilis, very rare now
Clinical	1. Portal cirrhosis 2. Bronze diabetes	Severe CHF Constrictive pericarditis	Tertiary syphilis Usually cardiovascular or CNS syphilis present
Pathology	Cirrhosis identical to fatty nutritional except: 1. Hemosiderin 4+ 2. Chocolate brown color to liver 3. No significant fat present in liver	Reversed portal cirrhosis with scars running between central vein areas instead of between portal triads	Consists of a gumma with granulomatous liver and large irregular areas of SCAR

CLINICAL PATHOLOGICAL CORRELATIONS IN CIRRHOSIS

Signs and Symptoms Due to Abnormal Bilirubin Metabolism

1. *Jaundice,* stains elastic tissue first and last; pruritus, especially with biliary cirrhosis, due to bile salts
2. In babies with bilirubin over 20 mg.% (mostly indirect), can get kernicterus; damage to basal ganglia
3. Hepatorenal syndrome (bile casts, tubular necrosis in some cases)

Signs and Symptoms Due to Increased Portal Pressure

1. Esophageal varices, 2/3 of patients have this, most common cause of bleeding with cirrhosis (also varices in duodenum or jejuneum can be seen)
2. Hemorrhoids
3. Caput medusae, rare
4. Peptic ulcer, 3rd most common cause of GI bleeding with cirrhosis
5. Banti's syndrome (splenomegaly, hemorrhage, leukocytopenia, anemia)
6. Ascites

Signs and Symptoms Due to Other Metabolic Defects

1. Hepatic coma: due to excess ammonia in blood; flapping tremor
   Pathology: increased number and size of protoplasmic (Alzheimer Type II) astrocytes in cerebral cortex and paraventricular nuclei
2. Abnormal endocrine disturbances (estrogens)
   a. testicular atrophy
   b. gynecomastia
   c. spider nevi
3. Low serum albumin—edema; low prothrombin—bleeding
4. Cirrhotic glomerulosclerosis: BM deposits of gamma globulin, foot processes fused in 25% of portal cirrhosis cases
5. Anemia
   a. hemolytic burr cell anemia; burr cells in blood with high indirect bilirubin, (?) cell membrane defect
   b. megaloblastic anemia: folate deficiency

CIRRHOSIS AND DEATH

1. The 9th most common cause of death in the U.S.A.
2. Most common causes of death in people with cirrhosis:
    a. Liver failure (hepatic coma) 35% of cirrhotic deaths
    b. Massive GI bleeding (ulcers or esophageal varices) 25% of cirrhotic deaths
    c. Intermittent infections, pneumonia: 10% of cirrhotic deaths
    d. Rest die of causes not related to cirrhosis

17 Pancreas and Biliary System

CANCER OF THE GALLBLADDER

Key Words
1. Rare
2. Occurs most frequently in women (75% of cases)
3. Associated with cholelithiasis (90% of cases)
4. Over 90% are adenocarcinomas
5. Most commonly (65%) are infiltrative, scirrhous tumors with invasion of liver
6. Widespread metastases rare
7. Hopeless prognosis

CARCINOMA OF THE BILE DUCTS

1. Very rare, less common than gallbladder carcinoma
2. More common in males than in females
3. Location (order of frequency):
   a. Common bile duct, lower end
   b. Junction of cystic duct
   c. Hepatic duct
   d. Cystic ducts
   e. Preampullary
   f. Ampulla, rarest, but best cure of all locations; may get GIT bleeding early
4. All adenocarcinomas usually well-differentiated
5. All produce jaundice and high alkaline phosphatase early

Cholelithiasis

	Mixed Stones	Pure Cholesterol Stones	Pure Bilirubin Stones
Relative incidence	90% of stones	7%	3%
Composition	Calcium carbonate Cholesterol Calcium bilirubinate	Cholesterol, crystalline	Calcium bilirubinate
Etiology	Unknown, central nidus usually cholesterol	Abnormal cholesterol metabolism, hypercholesterolemia	Hyperbilirubinemia most commonly due to excess hemolysis of RBC's

(Continued on facing page)

Cholelithiasis *(continued)*

	Acute	Chronic
Color	Variegated, concentric, yellow-black	White-yellow, bluish white Jet black
Special features	If stones of any type are multifaceted, there is more than one stone	
Complications	1. Most common complication is a stone in common duct: biliary colic, obstructive jaundice, biliary cirrhosis, ascending cholangitis 2. Acute cholecystitis with rupture: bile peritonitis 3. Gastrocolic fistula: gallstone, ileus 4. Gallbladder cancer rare, but 90% associated with stones	
Notes	1. Very rarely can have pure calcium carbonate stones 2. 20% of gallstones are radiopaque 3. Approximately 50% of nonopaque gallstones are manifested only by non-visualization of gallbladder by cholecystography. 4. Incidence varies from 10 to 20% of general population	

Cholecystitis

	Acute	Chronic
Etiology	Obstruction with superimposed bacterial infection, most common organism is *E. coli*	Obstruction
	Stones present in 95% of cases	Stones present in 95% of cases
Clinical	Acute surgical abdomen	*4 F's* Female Fat Forty Flatulent Fatty food intolerance Abdominal pain with fatty meal
Pathology		
Gross	Enlarged, edematous mottled gallbladder—often with stones	Normal or small with fibrosis, SCARRED wall
Micro	Polys, cellulitis, edema, necrosis	SCAR, chronic inflammatory cells
Special variations	1. Empyema: filled with pus 2. Gangrenous: green-black color 3. Porcelain: healed with calcification	1. Hydrops, clear fluid, complete obstruction of cystic duct 2. Cholecystitis glandularis proliferans, extension of sinuses into wall
Complications	1. Rupture: bile peritonitis 2. Gastrocolic fistula	Passage of stone into common bile duct, obstructive cirrhosis

CARCINOMA OF PANCREAS

General
1. 99% arise from ducts; 1% arise from acini
2. Most common in older age group
3. Male:female ratio = 2:1
4. Trousseau's sign may be present, migratory thrombophlebitis (trypsin)

Special

	Head	Body	Tail
Relative occurrence	60%	30%	10%
Clinical	1. Courvoisier's law: large gallbladder with cancer 2. Painless jaundice	———— severe weight loss ———— ———— back pain ———— ———— jaundice uncommon ————	
Pathology			
Gross	Large head with few metastases	Large body with many metastases	Large tail with many metastases
Micro	All usually well-differentiated adenocarcinomas; sometimes difficult to be sure they are malignant (perineural lymphatic invasion is a helpful finding)		
Prognosis	Poor, best cure rate of all three	Hopeless	Hopeless

Pancreatitis

	Acute Hemorrhagic Pancreatitis	Chronic (Relapsing) Pancreatitis
Etiology	UNKNOWN, plethora of theories: 1. Common channel theory (Opie): spasm, stone; 60% of people have common channel 2. Others: allergic, autoimmune, trypsin	1. Unknown 2. Recurrent mild attacks of acute pancreatitis 3. "Smoldering" pancreatitis 4. Chronic alcoholism
Clinical	1. Acute onset of severe abdominal pain 2. Shock early 3. Must differentiate from surgical abdomen, operation on acute pancreas is "kiss of death," amylase, lipase, lab tests 4. Facial cyanosis 5. Blue abdomen (Cullen's sign)	1. Recurrent bouts of bellyaches, "rum belly" 2. Usually hard to diagnose, focal calcification on x-ray is best sign 3. Enzymes not helpful
Pathology		
Gross	Enlarged, swollen pancreas with chalky white precipitates (calcium soaps)	Small, firm pancreas

(Continued on facing page)

Pancreatitis *(continued)*

	Acute Hemorrhagic Pancreatitis	Chronic (Relapsing) Pancreatitis
Micro	Early: acute inflammation, necrosis, fat necrosis, ground glass cytoplasm, varying amounts of hemorrhage with blood vessel digestion Late: healing with SCAR, chronic pancreatitis	Few foci of acute inflammation, mostly fibrosis around acini (like cinnabar) with chronic granulomatous inflammation, pseudocysts are common sequelae
Special features	1. Prognosis: 15% mortality without operation 2. Nearly 100% mortality with operation	1. Prognosis good 2. Steatorrhea and diabetes are late complications

CYSTS OF THE PANCREAS: KEY WORDS

Pseudocysts

1. Most common cyst of pancreas
2. NO epithelial lining
3. NO connection with ducts
4. Usually in tail or body of pancreas
5. Fluid has high amylase content
6. Usually solitary; largest cysts of pancreas (about 20 cm. diameter)

Congenital

1. Usually associated with abnormal ductal development
2. May be part of von Hippel—Lindau disease
3. Usually large: up to 5 cm. diameter and multiple

Retention

1. Due to obstruction of pancreatic duct, have epithelial lining
2. Usually smaller than congenital cyst, usually multiple

Neoplastic

1. Rare
2. Part of cystadenocarcinoma of pancreas
3. Usually large (5–15 cm.) and solitary

Pancreatic Duct and Acini Dilation

1. Dilation of ducts and acini with intussuscepted material
2. Etiology unknown
3. Seen in order of frequency
   a. Uremia
   b. Gastric cancer
   c. Small intestine obstruction
   d. Ulcerative colitis

BETA-CELL TUMOR OF THE PANCREAS

Whipple's Triad (Must Be Present)

1. Symptoms of hypoglycemia induced by fasting
2. Fasting blood sugar below 50 mg.%
3. Relief of symptoms by glucose administration

Pathology

90% are single adenomas
10% are multiple adenomas
 5% are due to diffuse hyperplasia
10% are malignant and will metastasize

Gross

Size of a dime—to 5 cm. diameter

Micro

Usually well-differentiated and there is POOR correlation between morphology and behavior, most important sign of malignancy is vein invasion

Prognosis

Good

Other Causes of Hypoglycemia

1. Long fasting
2. Idiopathic, probably most common cause
3. Liver disease, glycogenesis
4. Insulin-secreting tumors
5. Fibrosarcoma, bronchiogenic carcinoma

OTHER PANCREATIC ENDOCRINE SYNDROMES

1. Zollinger-Ellison syndrome; non-insulin-secreting tumor of pancreas (see Special Small Bowel Syndromes, Chap. 13), may be part of MEA I complex
2. Multiple endocrine adenopathies, Type I (MEA I)
   As part of this syndrome, patients may have insulin-, gastrin-, or glucagon-secreting adenomas of the pancreatic islets. They also can have adenomas of the pituitary, adrenal cortex, parathyroid and medullary cells of the thyroid. (See Chap. 19 for more complete discussion of MEA I)

18 Endocrine Glands I– Adrenals and Pituitary

ADRENAL GLAND

Resume of Structure and Function

Please see a clinical pathology or biochemistry book for details of steroid biochemistry.

Structure	Function
Cortex	
Zona glomerulosa (outer zone) (Stem cells (?) for other layers)	1. Secretes C-21 steroids, aldosterone and deoxycorticosterone, mineralocorticoids 2. Undergoes hyperplasia (focal) in Conn's syndrome
Zona fasciculata (middle and largest zone)	Secretes glucocorticoids, C-21 steroids (hydrocortisone, cortisone) Stores precursors of steroids
Zona reticularis (inner zone; thought to represent androgenic X zone in fetus)	1. Secretes sex hormones 2. C-19 steroids, androgens, testosterone, dehydroepiandrosterone, 17-ketosteroids 3. C-18 estrogens, estradiol, estriol, estrone
Medulla	
Large ovoid cords of chromaffin cells secreting epinephrine and norepinephrine, preformed hormone is stored	1. Vasoconstriction 2. Cardiotropic 3. Diabetogenic 4. Diagnose tumors by VMA, HVA, metanephrines, and catecholamine analysis on urine

Significant Tumors of the Adrenal Medulla

	Pheochromocytoma	Neuroblastoma and Related Tumors
Origin	From pheochromocytes, catecholamine-secreting chromaffin tissue (90% in adrenals)	From neuroblasts of chromaffin tissue
Clinical	1. Paroxysmal hypertension in adults; usually sustained in children 2. Most common in adults age 30–50, male and female equal 3. 5% associated with neurofibromas, von Hippel-Lindau's disease, or thyroid medullary carcinoma (MEA II) 4. Dx with regitine test (hypotensive), VMA, catecholamines and metanephrines in urine	1. *Adults* (very rare) usually benign 2. Sympathoblastoma (immature cells) Ganglioneuroma (mature cells) 3. *Children* (rare) neuroblastoma highly malignant lesion; may mature spontaneously to a ganglioneuroblastoma (both elements), then to ganglioneuroma (ganglion cells)—benign
Pathology		
Gross	Large hemorrhagic adrenal to 2000 g. (Average weight 100 g.)	Large, soft lobular, with foci of hemorrhage
Micro	Vascular channels, sinusoids lined with cells with granular cytoplasm Benign cells are pleomorphic	Neuroblastoma: small, round, lymphocyte-like cells, frequently with rosettes and pseudorosettes *Others:* ganglion cells with varying other cells present Ganglioneuroblastoma: cobweb network between cell masses
Special	1. Occurring outside adrenal chromaffin tissue, organ of Zuckerkandl most common extraadrenal site (7% of pheochromocytomas) 2. Bilateral (30% of pheochromocytomas) 3. Malignant with metastases (1% of pheochromocytomas) 4. Extraadrenal pheochromocytomas often have normetanephrine as predominant catecholamine	1. Prognosis improved with ganglion cells present 2. 40% of neuroblastomas are adrenal in origin 3. 10% of neuroblastomas are hormonally active with hormones similar to pheochromocytomas, especially homovanillic acid (HVA). HVA usually normal in pheochromocytomas 4. Neuroblastoma: MICRO identical to Ewing's tumor, retinoblastoma and medulloblastoma

Common Hyperadrenal Steroid Endocrinopathies

	Cushing's Syndrome	Adrenogenital Syndrome	Primary Hyperaldosteronism (Conn's Syndrome)
Definition	Hypertension, buffalo hump, obesity, hypokalemia, hypernatremia, abdominal striae and osteoporosis	Virilism with or without salt-losing crises and hypertension	Syndrome with hypertension, hypernatremia, hypokalemia, and polydipsia

Etiology	*Order of Frequency*
	1. External corticosteroids (iatrogenic)
	2. Cortical hyperplasia (70%)
	3. Adrenocortical adenoma (15%)
	4. Adreno-adenocarcinoma (10%)
	5. Extraadrenal tumors
	  a. pituitary adenoma, basophils
	  b. carcinoma of lung, breast, prostate, and others
		Lack of 21 hydroxylase (salt-losing), or 11 hydroxylase (hypertensive) enzymes	Excess aldosterone production
			Rarely can have similar syndrome due to nonaldosterone mineralocorticoid production (e.g., deoxycorticosterone, deoxycortisone)

Clinical	1. Syndrome as above
	2. Most common in adult women
		1. 85% in (XX) females: 50% under age 12, big phallus with female internal organs, female pseudohermaphrodites
		2. Young male: "little Hercules," precocious puberty, vomiting, salt-losing crisis
		3. Menstrual female: amenorrhea + masculinization, premature closure of epiphyses in all
			1. Syndrome as above, also
			  a. periodic paralysis
			  b. edema may occur
			2. Usually in young to middle-age

Pathology			
Gross	Normal or slightly enlarged gland, or adenoma, or carcinoma	Large gland 1. *Most* common: hyperplasia of adrenal 2. 2nd most common: cortical carcinoma 3. 3rd most common: cortical adenoma	Most commonly an adenoma of adrenal, rarely carcinoma or hyperplasia

(Continued on overleaf)

Common Hyperadrenal Steroid Endocrinopathies *(continued)*

	Cushing's Syndrome	*Adrenogenital Syndrome*	*Primary Hyperaldosteronism (Conn's Syndrome)*
Micro	Hyperplasia of zona fasciculata, adenoma or carcinoma, perinuclear hyaline degeneration in pituitary basophils due to excess corticosteroids (Crooke's hyaline degeneration)	Tumor cells have zona reticularis-like granules	Adenoma: zona glomerulosa-like cells is most common finding
Special features	Diagnose with 17-hydroxycortico-steroids in urine	1. Some tumors produce feminization 2. Ovarian tumors also may virilize or feminize 3. Diagnose with 17-ketosteroids in urine suppressed by cortisol	1. In children, usually have hyperplasia 2. Pinealoma produces secondary aldosteronism only in animals 3. Diagnose with serum aldosterone and renin evaluation

Hypoadrenal Steroid Endocrinopathies

	Adult Destructive Adrenal Lesion (Addison's Disease)	*Other Causes*
Etiology	Lack of corticosteroids—(?) autoimmune	*Iatrogenic atrophy*
Clinical	1. Weight loss (anorexia) 2. Hypotension 3. Hyperkalemia—hyponatremia 4. High plasma ACTH and MSH (skin pigmentation with melanin)	1. Due to excessively prolonged corticosteroid administration 2. Acute adrenal insufficiency when steroids are stopped
Pathology and pathogenesis	Order of frequency 1. Most common: idiopathic atrophy of adrenals, replaced by fat, anti-adrenal-cortical-cell antibody by FA 2. Infections: TBC most common 3. Bilateral metastases: lung most common primary 4. Hemorrhage: sepsis with vascular disease (Waterhouse-Friderichsen)—DIC 5. Surgical removal 6. Amyloidosis	*Congenital Adrenal Hypoplasia* 1. Anencephalic type: no X zone (same as seen in anencephalic monster) 2. Cytomegalic type: presence of large cells with eosinophilic cytoplasm as in cytomegalic inclusion disease

(Continued on opposite page)

Hypoadrenal Steroid Endocrinopathies *(continued)*

	Adult Destructive Adrenal Lesion (Addison's Disease)	*Other Causes*
Special comments	1. Strictly speaking Addison's disease as originally described by Addison was most commonly due to TBC (2nd most common cause idiopathic) 2. ALSO now may have toxic adrenal necrosis secondary to para-DDD (insecticide)	

PITUITARY
Diabetes Insipidus

Etiology

1. Most common cases due to secondary tumors involving midbrain or pituitary
2. 1/3 idiopathic, no anatomic lesion
3. Primary tumors of posterior are ultra-rare and are gliomas, NOT epithelial tumors

Diagnosis

By low osmolality of urine (cAMP normal). No cAMP in pseudodiabetes insipidus

Symptoms

Polyuria and polydypsia without glycosuria

Key Words

1. Very rare disease
2. Due to lack of ADH

Anterior Pituitary Hypofunction Syndromes

	Sheehan's Syndrome (Postpartum Necrosis)	*Simmonds' Cachexia (Panhypopituitarism)*
Etiology	Infarction of pituitary after or at delivery Rarely other causes (e.g., vascular thrombosis) Very rare in men	Idiopathic necrosis and SCARRING of pituitary, very rare Male:female ratio 1:2; no history of pregnancy
Clinical	Rare disease, usually with extensive hemorrhage and hypovolemic shock at delivery, and panhypopituitarism few weeks after delivery, death may occur	Rare, children, pituitary dwarfs (symmetrical) Adults, hypoendocrine syndromes (e.g., Addison's disease, myxedema, sterility, etc.)
Pathology	*Focal* necrosis continuing to scarring of pituitary	*Diffuse* necrosis continuing to fibrosis of pituitary
Special features	1. Posterior pituitary gland rarely affected 2. Most common cause of panhypopituitarism in adults 3. Chromophobe adenoma 2nd most common cause 4. Craniopharyngioma 3rd most common cause	1. Atrophy of all endocrine organs 2. Lab test for FSH easiest 3. Aldosterone normal, not under pituitary control 4. Can evaluate ACTH, TSH, GH, by RIA

Anterior Pituitary Adenomas*

	Basophil	*Acidophil*	*Chromophobe*
Relative percentage	3%	6%	91%
Function	Secretes TSH, ACTH, LATS, MSH(?), FSH, LH	Secretes growth hormone	(Reserve cell ?) ? Some may be functional
Symptoms	Causes less than 10% of Cushing's syndrome Rare cause of hypothyroidism	Gigantism in children Acromegaly in adults Visual Sx unusual	Visual field symptoms: bitemporal hemianopsia
Pathology			
Size	Usually microscopic	Semimicroscopic	Up to several centimeters
Micro	Masses of basophils, Crooke's hyaline change with Cushing's syndrome	Masses of acidophils	Chromophobes, no granules on EM
Special features	1. All tumors may occasionally show atypical staining cells and a mixed cell population is not uncommon 2. For all practical purposes, these tumors NEVER become malignant		

*Together these are the most common primary tumors of the pituitary

NONENDOCRINE TUMORS PRODUCING EXCESSIVE HORMONE EFFECTS

Antidiuretic Effect (ADH)

1. Carcinomas
   a. lung
      1) oat cell**
      2) squamous*
   b. pancreas
   c. duodenum
   d. thymus
2. Brain neoplasms
   a. various brain tumors
   b. cerebral carcinomatous metastases
   c. lymphosarcoma
   d. chromophobe adenoma

Chorionic Gonadotropic Effect

1. Placental tumor, benign or malignant (most common)**
2. Tumor of the testes, usually choriocarcinoma**
3. Malignant hepatoma
4. Adrenocortical carcinoma
5. Melanoma

Corticotropin Effect (ACTH)

1. Carcinomas
   a. lung
      1) oat cell
      2) squamous**
   b. thymus*
   c. pancreas
   d. prostate
   e. ovary
   f. parotid
   g. thyroid
   h. kidney
   i. stomach
   j. colon

Hypercalcemic Effect (Parathyroid Hormone-like)

1. Carcinomas
   a. lung, usually oat cell**
   b. breast**
2. Lymphomas
3. Sarcomas
4. Leukemias

Hypoglycemic Effect (Insulin-like)

1. Mesodermal tumors
   a. sarcomas

---

*significant incidence
**high incidence

      1) fibrosarcoma
      2) spindle cell carcinoma
      3) rhabdomyosarcoma
      4) leiomyosarcoma
      5) liposarcoma
      6) hemangiopericytoma
      7) neurofibrosarcoma
      8) Wilms' tumor
   b. fibromas*
2. Carcinomas
   a. liver
   b. stomach
   c. colon
   d. adrenals
   e. lung

Polycythemic Effect (Erythropoietin-like)

1. Renal lesions
   a. carcinomas (clear cell)**
   b. sarcoma
   c. benign adenoma
2. Uterine fibroma
3. Carcinomas
   a. liver*
   b. prostate
   c. stomach
   d. lung
   e. breast
4. Pheochromocytoma
5. Melanoma
6. Cerebellar hemangioblastoma

---

*significant incidence
**high incidence

19 Endocrine Glands II– Parathyroid and Thyroid

Parathyroid Glands

Primary Hyperparathyroidism	Secondary Hyperparathyroidism	Hypoparathyroidism
1. Most common cause: adenoma (85–90%; chief cells or mixed cells) 2. Second most common cause: wasserhelle cell hyperplasia (5–10%) 3. Get hypercalcemia and hypophosphatemia, loss of lamina dura of teeth; get band keratopathy in Bowman's membrane of cornea, also osteitis fibrosa cystica 4. Alkaline phosphatase normal early, elevated late	1. *Most* common type of hyperparathyroidism 2. Usually secondary to chronic renal disease (phosphate retention) 3. Osteitis fibrosa cystica (von Recklinghausen's disease of bone) 4. Chief cell hyperplasia, MOST common lesion in parathyroid gland	1. Most often iatrogenic 2. Tetany (Chvostek's sign) due to low serum calcium

THYROID GLAND

Benign Thyroid Tumors

Adenoma is MOST common
a. follicular: with glands; follicular adenoma is most common
b. Hürthle cell adenomas rarest
c. "C"-cell hyperplasia ("adenoma")—calcitonin secretion

Malignant Thyroid Tumors

1. Etiologic factors
   a. Radiation of head and neck
   b. ? excess TSH stimulation
2. Papillary carcinoma is MOST common, good prognosis, psammoma bodies
3. Other malignant tumors:
   a. follicular: with follicles
   b. anaplastic: poorest prognosis
   c. medullary: solid cords of "C" cells, usually with amyloid in stroma; associated with calcitonin secretion; have hypocalcemia

Goiter*

	Multiple Adenomatous Colloid Goiter (MACG)	Hyperthyroidism— Graves' Disease (Exophthalmic Goiter)	Simple Colloid Goiter
Etiology	Unknown	Excess T4, exophthalmos due to long-acting thyroid stimulator (LATS)—due to an immunoglobulin	Iodine deficiency
Clinical	Most common Young females 6 : 1 Iodine deficiency	Patients *hyperthyroid*, bug-eyed, hyperactive, nervous, T4, PBI, etc. high, usually females	Without thyroid symptoms Females more common than males
Gross	Asymmetrically enlarged gland, largest thyroid	Gland—large, meaty, symmetrical, hemorrhagic	Nodular, symmetrical, enlarged gland
Micro	Large, colloid-filled follicles, flattened cells, hemorrhage + calcification often seen	Papillary formation, scalloped follicles Tall, columnar cells All treated with Lugol's solution (iodides) to cause colloid storage and devascularization, propylthiouracil produces hyperplasia of follicles and blocks organification of iodide	Large follicles with flattened cells
Lab	PBI, T4, etc., usually normal; TSH sometimes increased	PBI, T4, etc., elevated; TSH may be decreased or normal	Normal or slightly low T4 or PBI; TSH is normal or elevated

*Goiter=enlarged thyroid, over 20 g. due to any cause

Hypothyroidism

Cretinism: hypothyroid at birth, most commonly due to thyroid aplasia; dwarf, mentally retarded; must be diagnosed early to prevent permanent brain damage and MR

Dyshormonogenesis (goiter) syndromes: besides classic cretinism, there are at least five congenital, hereditary dyshormonogenesis syndromes, with low or abnormal iodinated compounds in the blood. (See HBCP, Chap. 9.)

Myxedema: hypothyroidism in adult, low PBI and T4, thick skin, coarse hair, slow, lethargic, thyroid atrophic; most common cause is idiopathic atrophy

Thyroid Diseases of Unknown Etiology

	Subacute Thyroiditis	*Hashimoto's Disease*	*Riedel's Struma*
Etiology	(?)	Autoimmune (?) 97% have high ATA titers	? Burned-out Hashimoto's
Gross	Slight, asymmetric enlargement	Tan-brown color, symmetrical enlargement	Small, asymmetric, hard, fibrous thyroid
Micro	Giant cells, granulomas	1. Lymphoid follicle, lymphoid infiltrates 2. Microfollicles (glands) 3. Hurthle cell metaplasia	Fibrous tissue with rare epithelial cells
Special features		Also called lymphoepithelial goiter and struma lymphomatosa	May mistake for cancer on gross

Relative Incidence of Carcinoma of the Thyroid

Papillary adenocarcinoma 46%
Solid and follicular adenocarcinoma 26%
Giant cell carcinoma 13%
Hurthle cell carcinoma 9%
Unclassified carcinomas including medullary 6%

PARATHORMONE

1. Secreted by parathyroid glands
2. Regulates calcium and phosphate metabolism and increases
   a. calcium absorption from GIT
   b. tubular resorption of calcium
   c. tubular secretion of phosphate
   d. the release of calcium and phosphate from bone
3. Causes bone resorption
4. Low serum calcium causes parathormone to be produced

CALCITONIN

1. Secreted by "C" or parafollicular cells of the thyroid gland, not by parathyroid gland
2. Prevents excess hypercalcemic response to parathormone by preventing greater than physiologic amounts of calcium from leaving bone
3. Prevent bone resorption
4. Causes increased sodium and water excretion by kidney
5. Carcinoma and "C"-cell hyperplasia of thyroid are associated with increased calcitonin levels

MEA SYNDROMES
MULTIPLE ENDOCRINE ADENOMAS (ADENOMATOSES) (MEA)

General

1. There are currently recognized two MEA syndromes with some distinct and some overlapping patterns of endocrine adenomas and other findings.
2. The etiologies of these MEA syndromes are currently thought to be autosomal dominant with poor penetrance.
3. Any individual patient may have a full-blown syndrome or a *forme fruste* with only partial expression of the syndrome.
4. In general medical practice these syndromes are uncommon to rare in occurrence. The currently defined MEA syndromes are summarized in the following table.

Summary of Components of Multiple Endocrine Adenomatoses Syndromes

Involved Organ	MEA I (Wermer's Syndrome)	MEA II (Sipple's Syndrome)
Thyroid—(medullary carcinoma or hyperplasia)	Common	Very common
Parathyroid adenomas	Very common	Common
Adrenal cortex adenomas	Very common	Common
Pituitary adenomas	Very common	NOT seen
Pheochromocytomas	NOT seen	Very common
Pancreas (insulin or non-insulin producing adenomas)	Very common	NOT seen
Peptic ulcers (Z-E pattern frequent)	Very common	NOT seen
Neuromas, especially on mucous membranes	NOT seen	Very common

20 Kidney– Glomerular Diseases

GLOMERULUS

Endothelial Cell

1. Lines capillaries of glomerulus
2. Swells and proliferates in disease

Basement Membrane of Endothelial Cell

1. Glycoprotein central dense area (lamina densa); and lighter area (lamina rara) on each side (externa and interna)
2. Normally about 3000 Å thick; thickened in many diseases (lose protein with basement membrane damage)

Epithelial Cell

1. Covers capillary and forms visceral layer of Bowman's capsule
2. Foot processes abut on basement membrane (BM)
3. Foot processes lost or fused in many diseases

Mesangial Cell (Deep Endothelial Cell)

1. Cell of stalk, mesangium, or axial region
2. Mesenchymal cell—totipotential (?)
3. Functions: supportive, phagocytic
4. May be modified endothelial cell: often confused with endothelial cell
5. Proliferates in many disease states

JUXTAGLOMERULAR APPARATUS

STRUCTURE

Macula Densa

1. Special concentration of tubular epithelial cells at junction of loop of Henle and distal convoluted tubule
2. High concentration of acid mucopolysaccharide in cells
3. NO BM in macula densa area

Juxtaglomerular Body (Juxtaglomerular Cells; JG)

1. Group of modified smooth muscle cells resembling epithelioid cells, in media of *afferent* arteriole, just before entering glomerulus, in contact with macula densa
2. Cell contains granules-renin (?)

3. Cell contains myofilaments
4. Adrenergic nerves abut on JG cells

Polkissen (Polar Pad)

1. Group of small cells with pale nuclei between macula densa and JG body
2. Function unknown

FUNCTION

Renin is trophic, via angiotensin system, to aldosterone (zona glomerulosa of adrenal)
Causes sodium retention and potassium loss.
Inverse relationship between number of granules in JG cells and serum sodium levels
Can get excess JG granules by sodium restriction or partial occlusion of renal artery
Increased granules may be seen in some, but not all, cases of hypertension

GLOMERULONEPHRITIS (GN)

There currently are thought to be two immunological mechanisms for glomerulonephritis. They are immune complex disease and anti-basement membrane antibody glomerulonephritis.

IMMUNE COMPLEX DISEASE

In this disease circulating, non-precipitating, non-antiglomerular basement membrane antigen-antibody complex (non-AGBMA) formed in antigen excess is deposited on the basement membranes with the activation of complement and the chemotactic attraction of WBC's and the subsequent release of lysosomal enzymes and inflammation and/or other changes characteristic of non-AGBMA immune complex disease.

Morphologic Characteristics

Light microscope: Proliferation (poststreptococcal GN) or no proliferation (membranous GN) of glomerular cells
Fluorescent antibody: Lumpy, bumpy, granular deposits consisting of IgG as well as complement (especially C_3). Other immunoglobulins may be seen.
Electron microscope: Subepithelial epimembranous lumpy deposits with fused or absent epithelial foot processes

Renal Diseases Currently Considered to Be Due to Immune Complexes

1. Poststreptococcal GN: most common and classic
2. Lupus erythematosus GN (focal membranous): EM deposits are classically subendothelial as well as subepithelial. (The presence of "fingerprints" or organized viral capsid-like material within the immune complexes is said to be diagnostic of lupus erythematosus on EM.)
3. Polyarteritis nodosa: Wegener's granulomatosis GN
4. Anaphylactoid purpura GN
5. Serum sickness GN
6. Membranous GN
7. Membranoproliferative GN (hypocomplementemic GN): Some consider it a variant of poststreptococcal GN, others consider it a separate entity

ANTIGLOMERULAR BASEMENT MEMBRANE ANTIBODY GLOMERULONEPHRITIS (AGBMA-GN)

This is currently thought to be due to the reaction of circulating antiglomerular basement membrane antibodies (AGBMA) with the subsequent attachment and activation of complement and chemotaxis and activation of WBC's with membrane and glomerular inflammation and destruction.

Morphologic Characteristics

Light microscope: Usually causes proliferation of glomerular cells, frequently with crescent formation

Fluorescent antibody: Smooth linear FA deposits of IgG, with or without other immunoglobulins, and complement (especially C_3) along basement membrane. Fibrinogen, if present, is usually focal, not linear, in distribution.

Electron microscope: "Linear" epimembranous and intramembranous deposits of electron-dense material with loss or fusion of foot processes of epithelial cells

Renal Diseases Currently Considered to Be Exclusively or Frequently Due to AGBMA

1. Goodpasture's syndrome: By definition all cases have AGBMA
2. Rapidly progressive GN with crescent formation: most, but *not* all, cases found to be AGBMA in etiology
3. There are many experimental models of AGBMA GN in animals.

GOODPASTURE'S SYNDROME

Etiology

1. AGBMA to renal and pulmonary basement membranes

Clinical Features

1. Pulmonary hemorrhage with pulmonary symptoms
2. Hematuria, proteinuria; rapid renal failure

Pathology

Gross: Same as poststreptococcal or rapidly progressive GN
Micro: Kidney: usually like subacute GN with proliferation and crescents
Lungs: Intraalveolar hemorrhage, heart failure cells, alveolar wall thickening and necrosis

Fluorescent Antibody

Diffuse, smooth, linear, ribbon-like IgG, with or without other immunoglobulins with complement in renal and pulmonary BM

EM

Smooth, linear, epimembranous and intramembranous deposits with fusion or loss of foot processes

RX

Not responsive to steroids; often RXed by nephrectomy and transplants

ACUTE POSTSTREPTOCOCCAL (PROLIFERATIVE) GLOMERULONEPHRITIS

Etiology

Post-group A beta-hemolytic streptococcal infection, especially Types 4, 12, 25, and Red Lake, also other foreign antigens

Pathogenesis

Altered immunity to streptococcus (?) or other antigens; IgG with or without other immunoglobulins, complement, and antigen deposits; focal, lumpy, on epithelial surface of BM; C_3, C_5, and ($C_{5,6,7}$ complex) are chemotactic for WBC's

Classical Clinical Features

1. MOST common in children; 85% to 95% recover, 1% to 3% die, 1% to 2% develop rapidly progressive GN
2. Adults only: 60% recover, rest develop chronic renal disease or die in acute phase

Classic Signs and Symptoms

1. Back pain
2. Fever
3. Slight or no edema
4. Slight to moderate blood pressure elevation
5. Many RBC's in urine (smoky urine); RBC casts in urine
6. Oliguria
7. Slight albuminuria (milligram amounts)
8. BUN normal or slight elevation

Gross

1. Large, congested kidney, rarely with petechiae on surface
2. Bulging cut surface, sometimes with petechiae
3. Capsule strips with ease
4. Smooth external surface

Micro

EXUDATION early with PROLIFERATION later
1. Swollen endothelial cells (relatively bloodless glomeruli), proliferation later
2. Collections of neutrophils, exudative in glomeruli early
3. *Lobular* stalk thickening, mesangial and endothelial cell proliferation ($>$ 50 cells per glomerulus)
4. Tubular (?) degeneration

FA

1. Lumpy "granular" deposits with IgG and C_3 along BM and in mesangium
2. Focal fibrinogen deposits also frequent

EM

1. Slight thickening of BM
2. *Focal,* lumpy, electron-dense deposits, classically on epithelial side of BM
3. Fused or absent epithelial foot processes

RAPIDLY PROGRESSIVE (SUBACUTE, CRESCENTIC) GLOMERULONEPHRITIS

Etiology

1. Most cases idiopathic
2. May be secondary to acute poststreptococcal glomerulonephritis or other immune complexes, or AGBMA disease

Pathogenesis

Immune complex disease or AGBMA disease with fibrinogen deposits

Classical Clinical Features

1. Early findings similar to acute GN
2. Most progress to renal failure and uremia, with or without passing through nephrotic syndrome

Classic Signs and Symptoms

NEPHROTIC SYNDROME consisting of:
1. Anasarca (generalized edema)
2. Albuminuria, massive, up to 8 g./24 hr.
3. Hypoalbuminemia with reversed A/G ratio
4. Hypercholesterolemia
5. BUN NORMAL or very slightly elevated (not over 35 mg.%)
6. Basal metabolism low, loss of T4-binding protein
7. Slight or no hypertension
8. Hyaline casts, oval fat bodies, and Maltese crosses in urine

Gross

1. Large pale kidney; capsule strips easily
2. Smooth external surface, bulging cut surface

Micro

1. Key features: proliferation of epithelial cells with crescent formation
2. *Epithelial crescents:* adhesions of capillary tuft to Bowman's capsule
3. Epithelial, mesangial, and endothelial proliferation
4. Proliferation of proximal convoluted tubule cells "increscents"
5. Tubule cells, cloudy swelling, fat vacuoles, Maltese crosses (cholesterol esters) in urine

FA

1. Lumpy, "granular" BM and mesangial deposits in immune complex types
2. Linear, smooth BM deposits in AGBMA types

EM

1. In immune complex type: basement membrane diffusely thickened, lumpy epimembranous deposit, fused or absent foot processes
2. In AGBMA type: linear, intramembranous, and epimembranous deposits with fusion and loss of foot processes

Notes

1. Not all cases are rapidly progressive; some show acute onset
2. The second most common cause of nephrotic syndrome in children, third most common cause of nephrotic syndrome in adults

CHRONIC GLOMERULONEPHRITIS

Etiology

1. Poststreptococcal glomerulonephritis
2. Membranous glomerulonephritis
3. Idiopathic

Pathogenesis

Scarring: USUALLY from preexisting immune complex or AGBMA disease; often cannot tell cause, END-STAGE KIDNEY

Clinical Features

USUALLY in older children or young adults; none recover

Classic Signs and Symptoms

1. Renal failure + uremia
2. Small amount of albumin in urine
3. Anasarca lost
4. BUN, creatinine, phosphorus, potassium rise—high
5. Blood pressure rises
6. Specific gravity of urine becomes FIXED at 1.010; broad casts in urine
7. Hypocalcemia, secondary hyperparathyroidism

Gross

1. Small contracted kidney, big heart (kidneys may fit in left ventricle)
2. Granular surface, like nephrosclerosis but granules are larger and kidneys smaller
3. Capsule adherent, strips with difficulty

Micro

ALL glomeruli hyalinized, many fine fibrous SCARS, tubules atrophic, hyalinized arterioles and arterials, END-STAGE KIDNEY

EM & FA

EM & FA patterns confusing; can see either immune complex or AGBMA pattern

Membranous Glomerulonephritis vs. Lipoid Nephrosis

	Idiopathic Membranous (Transmembranous) Glomerulonephritis	Lipoid Nephrosis "Foot Process Disease"
Etiology	1. Unknown 2. Altered immunity (e.g., gold)	1. Unknown 2. NO visible antibodies to or on BM
Pathogenesis	Immune complex deposits: IgG, antigen, complement; tactic for polys 50% are normocomplementemic 50% are hypocomplementemic	Totally unknown Foot processes FUSED No antibody deposits Fat-positive tubular cells
Clinical	1. Insidious onset; *usually* no history of streptococcal or other infections 2. Most common in young adults 3. Only about 15% recover	1. Lipoid most common cause of nephrotic syndrome in children; second most common cause in adults

(Continued on facing page)

Membrane Glomerulonephritis vs. Lipoid Nephrosis *(continued)*

	Idiopathic Membranous (Transmembranous) Glomerulonephritis	*Lipoid Nephrosis "Foot Process Disease"*
	4. Nephrotic syndrome with gradual progression to chronic renal failure 5. Most common cause of nephrotic syndrome in adults	2. Usually explosive onset with nephrotic syndrome 3. Most common in children, rare in adults 4. Prognosis is good; well over 50% recover with steroid RX 5. Death usually due to infection, (hypogammaglobulinemia frequent)
Gross	1. Large, pale kidney 2. Capsule strips with ease 3. Slight bulge to cut surface	1. Large, pale kidney 2. Capsule strips with ease 3. Slight bulge to cut surface
Micro	No proliferation of renal glomerular cells	No visible changes of BM on H & E section
Early	Focal epimembranous, argyrophilic deposits (spikes) with methenamine silver stain	No proliferation of renal glomerular cells
Intermediate	Smooth thickening of BM on H&E, without proliferation. "Tram-track" phenomenon: nonargyrophilic centers with argyrophilia on both sides of BM with methenamine silver stain	Normal or slight diffuse thickening of BM with marked lipid deposit (cholesterol esters) in proximal convoluted tubules (lipoid nephrosis); no proliferation
Late	Generalized nonargyrophilia of basement membranes	Same as classic or within normal limits
FA	Lumpy "granular" BM deposits in immune complex pattern	No ag-ab or complement deposits
EM	*Note:* Proliferation is NOT a prominent feature Lumpy, bumpy, epimembranous deposits with moderate to marked fusion and loss of foot processes. BM spikes protrude between complex deposits	Fusion of foot processes with NO endo- or epimembranous deposits ("foot PROCESS disease")
Urine	Oval fat bodies Maltese crosses (cholesterol esters), 1+ to 2+ Hyaline casts, 1+ to 3+	Oval fat bodies and Maltese crosses, 4+ Hyaline casts, 1+ to 3+

21 Kidney–Tubular and Interstitial Diseases

Pyelonephritis

	Acute	Chronic
Etiology	*E. coli,* others—coliform, staphylococcus	
Pathogenesis	1. Ascending, USUALLY with OBSTRUCTION 2. BPH in males 3. Honeymoon cystitis and pregnancy in females, on right more than left	
Clinical features	1. Pyuria: over 100,000 bacteria/ml. in urine is *significant* bacteriuria 2. Back pain, fever in acute pyelonephritis 3. MOST common complication: hypertension	
Gross	Asymmetrical lesion	Asymmetrical lesion
Size	Normal or slightly enlarged kidneys	Small irregular kidney
Surface	White nodules ringed with red	Irregular U-shaped scars
Cut surface	White, linear lesion with red around columns of Bertin	Small, scarred kidney, U-shaped scars usually *do not* extend to medulla; blunted calyces
Micro	Polys, necrosis, abscesses, suppuration	1. *Peri*glomerular fibrosis 2. Dilatation of tubules with hyaline casts (thyroidization) 3. Interstitial fibrosis 4. Chronic inflammatory cells
Urine	Glitter cells (activated polys), 3+ to 4 + WBC casts, 4+ Granular casts, not broad casts	Glitter cells, 1 to 2+ WBC, broad granular casts 2+
Prognosis	GOOD	POOR
Complications	1. Hypertension, metastatic abscesses, necrotizing papillitis (phenacetin, diabetes, pyelonephritis) 2. Suspected reasons why medulla is more susceptible to infection than cortex: a. Poor blood supply b. High ammonia level inhibits C_4 component of complement. c. High osmolality inhibits WBC function, lets L forms of bacteria survive 3. Pyelonephritis is MOST common cause of clinically significant renal disease in some series (35% die of renal disease)	

Kidney in Hypertension

	Benign Nephrosclerosis	Malignant Nephrosclerosis
Gross	Granular surface (Morocco leather or pigskin) Symmetrical lesion	Flea-bitten kidney Symmetric lesion
Size	Small	Normal if purely malignant
Micro	1. Arteriolar nephrosclerosis Hyalinized afferent arterioles, hyalinized glomeruli 2. Arterial nephrosclerosis Hyalinized arcuate and intralobular arteries a. Hyalinized glomeruli b. Proliferation of intima (onionskin) c. Focal collections of lymphocytes and plasma cells in cortex	1. Hyalinized glomeruli 2. Proliferation of intima (onion skin) 3. Collection of lymphocytes and plasma cells in cortex 4. Fibrinoid NECROSIS of afferent arterioles is ONLY absolute morphological criterion 5. (1), (2), and (3) found only if benign nephrosclerosis is preexisting
Special notes	1. Only 5% die of renal failure; MOST common renal disease in patients over 50 years of age 2. These findings may be seen with arteriosclerosis without significant hypertension	1. 95% of untreated patients die of renal failure (uremia) 2. Only about 5% of all hypertensives develop malignant hypertension

Other Renal Lesions I

	Renal Vein Thrombosis Hypertension	Nephrosis (Toxemia) of Pregnancy	Amyloidosis
Etiology	Primary rare, USUALLY secondary to other renal diseases: 1. Membranous GN 2. Pyelonephritis 3. Amyloidosis	Pressor substance by placenta (?) Unknown	Secondary to: 1. TBC 2. Chronic osteomyelitis 3. Rheumatoid arthritis
Clinical	1. Nephrotic syndrome: gradual occlusion 2. Flank pain, hematuria, fever and leukocytosis =acute renal occlusion	Toxemia of pregnancy: Preeclampsia: (1) hypertension (2) edema (3) albuminuria Eclampsia: (1), (2), (3), with convulsions	Nephrotic syndrome to renal failure (uremia)
Gross	Acute: diffusely mottled kidney with no increase in size Chronic: large, pale kidney	Congested early Late: mottled kidneys, yellow and red, uric acid infarcts common	Large, pale kidneys waxy

(Continued on overleaf)

Other Renal Lesions I *(continued)*

	Renal Vein Thrombosis Hypertension	Nephrosis (Toxemia) of Pregnancy	Amyloidosis
Micro	Acute: necrosis, diffuse with tubular hemorrhage Chronic: 1. No proliferation of glomerular cells 2. Thickened basement membrane 3. Tubular atrophy 4. Tubular damage more than glomerular damage	1. *Edema* of all cells of glomerular tuft (MOST severe in endothelial cells) 2. Thickened basement membrane, smooth due to fibrin on endomembranous surface	Eosinophilic amyloid deposits in glomeruli; best stained with Congo red or crystal violet stains; apple-green birefringence with polarized light
FA	Granular BM deposits	$\pm$	Thioflavin T positive
EM	Lumpy, bumpy, *epi-*membranous deposits with fused and atrophic foot processes	*Endo*membranous fibrin deposits	Fibrillary deposits with 100Å periodicity in and around BM and in mesangium, mostly extracellular. Foot processes atrophic
Special comments	Most frequent underlying cause of renal vein thrombosis is idiopathic membranous glomerulonephritis; may be secondary to: a. CHF b. Constrictive pericarditis c. Inferior vena cava obstruction	May progress to renal cortical necrosis, especially if fibrin is present. Get thrombi in small vessels + necrosis + hemorrhage	Paramyloid may be present in multiple myeloma

INTERSTITIAL NEPHRITIS

Definition

Inflammation of kidney, primarily involving the interstitial areas

Acute

Often due to hypersensitivity to drugs. Penicillin, sulfonamides, and phenacetin are especially frequent causes, but at least 100 different drugs or other compounds can cause nephrotoxicity with acute interstitial nephritis. Also seen with some acute infections. Micro: interstitial edema, round cells, some polys, and, usually, eosinophils; sometimes with vasculitis. May resolve or progress to chronic interstitial nephritis

Chronic

May be seen with syphilis, TBC, or other chronic infections or from acute (above) Micro: round cells in interstitium with scarring. May have dilated tubules with thyroidization; may be impossible to distinguish morphologically from chronic pyelonephritis

Other Renal Lesions II

	Cholemic Nephrosis	*Myeloma Kidney*
Etiology	Liver failure: biliary obstruction, bile salts (?); shock (?): hemolysis, unconjugated bilirubin	Abnormal clone of plasma cells multiplies
Symptoms	No renal symptoms to renal failure and jaundice (hepatorenal syndrome?)	Same as multiple myeloma
Gross	Bile-stained kidney	Normal usually but may be scarred
Micro	Brown-green pigment casts in tubules, with or without necrosis of tubular epithelial cells	Casts, myeloma proteins in tubules; dilated tubules with rupture; giant cells and chronic inflammatory cells (granulomas) in interstitium; NO plasma cell infiltrates in kidney
Special comments	1. May have hepatorenal syndrome without morphologic renal damage 2. Alone, bile casts don't cause renal failure (?) 3. It is lower nephron nephrosis + renal failure or "hepatorenal" failure	Paramyloid: abnormal staining "amyloid" often associated

OTHER RENAL LESIONS III: KEY WORDS

de Toni-Fanconi Syndrome

1. Uncommon, hereditary
2. Aminoaciduria, glycosuria and hyperphosphaturia
3. Vitamin D-resistant rickets; no 1-hydroxylation of 25-hydroxycholecalciferol (Vitamin D_3 production)
4. "Swan-neck" deformity of renal tubules

Acute Cortical Necrosis

1. Shunting blood to medulla (Trueta?) (DIC ?)
2. MOST common in pregnancy
3. Can occur in severe infections
4. Mottled yellow-red kidney cortex
5. MICRO: focal hemorrhage and necrosis

Flea-Bitten Kidney

1. Malignant hypertension
2. Collagen-vascular diseases
3. Leukemias + lymphomas

Renal Infarct

1. End-artery circulation
2. V-shaped scars often extend to medulla

Benign Kidney Tumors (Most Common)

	Cortex	Medulla
Name	Renal cortical adenoma	Fibroma
Gross	Yellow, usually small All < 2 cm. in diameter	Small, white, firm tumor in medulla
Micro	Clear cells with pseudotubular and gland formation, identical to hypernephroma	Spindle cells, benign-looking
Note	1. If over 2 or 3 cm. in diameter, called a hypernephroma 2. Present in about 25% of all autopsies	Less common than cortical adenoma

Malignant Kidney Tumors

	Renal Cell Carcinoma (Hypernephroma)	Wilms' Tumor (Embryonal Mixed Tumor)
Incidence	80% of all malignant tumors of kidney Male 2: female 1 USUALLY in mid- or late-adult age group	Uncommon USUALLY in children under 10 years About 5% (higher in some series) of all malignant tumors of childhood
Signs and symptoms	MOST common presenting symptom-HEMATURIA: often silent until metastases appear	MOST common presenting symptom-ABDOMINAL MASS; pain and hematuria MAY occur
Gross	Large mass, dirty, red-brown, *hemorrhagic,* white, and > 3 cm. in diameter	Large, variegated tumor, 10%–20% bilateral
Micro	Several patterns: 1. Tubular adenocarcinoma 2. Clear cells (clear cell carcinoma) 3. Solid cords, many blood vessels	Abortive glomeruli Mesenchymatous area Spindle cells Striated muscle cells
Special notes	1. If < 3 cm. diameter, they are *adenomas* 2. Metastases commonly via renal vein; "cannonball" metastases in lung 3. 5-year survival 10%–35% depending on size of tumor	1. Probably a variant of rhabdomyosarcoma or mixed mesenchymal tumor (teratoma) 2. 10%–40% 5-year survival; sensitive to radiation and chemotherapy

UREMIA—RENAL FAILURE

Most Common Causes
1. Chronic pyelonephritis=most common cause in late childhood and old age
2. Proliferative and chronic glomerulonephritis=most common causes in ages 15 to 50
3. Benign nephrosclerosis (with or without malignant change) is a common cause in young and middle-aged adults

Clinical Manifestations

1. Skin: uremic frost USUALLY around mouth, pruritus, yellow, sallow pigmentation
2. Bone marrow: hypoplasia of erythrocytic series, toxic depression, ANEMIA, bleeding problems, abnormal platelets, decreased stickiness and Pf_3
3. Cardiovascular
   a. Fibrinous pericarditis
   b. Arrhythmias, potassium toxicity
4. Nervous system (CNS): twitching, convulsions, apathy, coma; (PNS): lower extremity hyperesthesia, axonal degeneration in sural nerve, deficiency of ionized calcium (?), cerebral edema
5. GI tract: esophagitis to colitis, acute inflammation and ulceration
6. Pancreas: dilated ducts and acini with inspissated material
7. Respiratory system: uremic interstitial pneumonitis, Kussmaul breathing
8. Eye grounds: vision loss, findings identical to retinal hypertension

Cystic Diseases of the Kidney

Simple or Solitary Cysts	Retention Cysts	Multilocular Cysts	Congenital Polycystic Kidneys (4 types)
Pathogenesis			
Tubular dilatation in vascular or inflammatory disease	Nephrosclerotic kidney disease	Unknown	Mostly hereditary
Incidence			
Common	Most common	Very rare	Uncommon
Age			
Adults	Adults	Any	Children (except Type III)
Laterality			
Usually unilateral	Usually bilateral	Usually unilateral	All bilateral except Type II
Gross			
Single or few cysts, usually cortical	Small blebs, clear fluid	Circumscribed multilocular cyst	Varies
Micro			
Nondescript lining	Flattened to cuboidal epithelium	Smooth muscle in capsule	Varies

Polycystic Kidney: Classification

Type (from Potter)	I	II	III	IV
	Dilatation and hyperplasia of collecting tubules	Inhibition of ureteral ampullary activity	Multiple abnormalities of development	Urethral or ureteral obstruction
	Proximal nephrons normal	Defective formation of collecting tubules	Like Type II, but less extensive	Cysts caused by obstruction—membranes
	(Polycystic disease, infantile type)	Blind end of collecting tubules become cystic	Many normal nephrons formed	Cysts, few, beneath capsule
	Spongy appearance	Failure of nephrogenesis	Some proximal nephrons cystic	Embryogenesis almost normal
	Small cysts	(Aplastic, hypoplastic kidney; multicystic disease; multilocular cyst)	(Polycystic disease, adult type)	(Obstructive uropathy with cystic kidney)
Pathogenesis	Hereditary	Congenital	Hereditary (dominant)	Congenital
Frequency	Rare	Relatively common	Most common	Rare
Age	Infants only	Infants, children, adults	Infants, children, adults	Infants
Laterality	Always bilateral	Usually unilateral; bilateral only in stillborn infants	Usually bilateral	Usually bilateral
Kidney size	Large	Large or normal	Large	Normal
Prognosis and special features	Bile ducts always cystic, death in infancy	Varies, may live long with partial involvement	Usually fatal in middle age	Varies with severity; usually fatal early

Type III Polycystic Kidney Disease

Associated conditions: Berry aneurysm
Cystic liver
Cystic pancreas
Hemangioma of brain

Death due to:
1. Uremia (1/3)
2. Hypertension (1/3)
3. Unrelated cause (1/3)

Tubular Diseases

	Lower Nephron Nephrosis	Toxic Nephrosis
Etiology	Shock, burns, trauma, severe hemorrhage Crush syndrome Intestinal obstruction Incompatible blood transfusion Blackwater fever, dehydration	Ingestion of toxic chemicals (mercury MOST common cause, also carbon tetrachloride, polymyxin, neomycin, and penthrane anesthesia)
Pathogenesis	Anoxia to tubule	Poisoning of tubule by chemicals (?) Precipitation of protein enzymes (?)
Symptoms	1. Early oliguria to anuria 2. Later azotemia 3. If recover, diuresis and electrolyte imbalance a problem	Same as lower nephron nephrosis
Gross	Yellow cortex, red outer 1/3 medulla	Similar to lower nephron nephrosis
Micro		
Early	1. Focal necrosis of tubules, mostly distal with casts 2. Casts: hyaline, waxy, granular, "brown sugar" 3. Dilatation of tubules 4. Extravasation into surrounding tissues with inflammation around tubules	1. Necrosis of proximal tubule cells (colloid droplets with Hg) 2. Tubular BM intact 3. Focal calcification
Later	Regeneration, mitotic figures, and loss of casts if healing takes place; BM loss	1. Morphology of regeneration similar to lower nephron nephrosis 2. Regeneration less common than in lower nephron nephrosis
Prognosis	Varies with underlying disease, but overall recovery about 50%	

22 Lower Genitourinary Including Newer Concepts

CONGENITAL ANOMALIES OF THE URETERS

Double Ureters

Partial or complete
If complete, double ureters are present; lower orifice in bladder is ALWAYS connected to upper renal segment

Ectopic Ureter

In males: enters posterior urethra proximal to external sphincter USUALLY through seminal vesicles
Hydronephrosis is MOST common complication
In females: total urinary incontinence with normal voiding, MAY exit anywhere along urethra

Megaloureter (in Children) Theories:

Neurogenic:
  Abnormal sympathetic and parasympathetic nerves, plexuses and fibers
  Frequently accompanies Hirschsprung's disease
Obstructive:
  Posterior urethral valves, hard to discover, USUALLY also has distended bladder with bladder neck obstruction
  With advanced lesion, get obstruction due to angulation

Postcaval Ureter (VERY RARE)

Obstructive uropathy
Key Words: mesial displacement of ureter with *S-shaped shadow* on IVP

Ureterocele

Ballooning of ureteral orifice into bladder lumen

Theory: persistent Chwalla's membrane blocking ureteral orifice; usually absorbed at term
Diagnosis: Cobra-head ureterovesical junction on IVP

CONGENITAL ANOMALIES OF THE URINARY BLADDER AND URETHRA

Patent urachus: failure of closure of allantoic duct (drainage of urine at umbilicus)

Urachal cyst: closure of both ends of duct; symptom—intermittent abdominal swelling

130

URINARY CALCULI (RENAL COLIC)

Etiology
Metabolic
1. Vitamin A deficiency (rat—experimental)
2. Hyperparathyroidism
3. Gout
4. Cystinuria (small crystals, renal calculi)
5. Recumbency, especially with bone injury, and demineralization

Local Factors
1. Stasis commonest factor in etiology
2. Urinary infection commonly associated with calculi, especially with urea-splitting bacteria, *Proteus vulgaris*
3. Colloids protect, increase solubility of crystals
4. Randall's plaque: calcified plaques at or near apex area of renal papillae may be source of calculi

Symptoms

1. Pain: intermittent CVA pain
2. Infection frequent with stone (90% radiopaque)
3. Hematuria

Types of Stones

MOST common type (in either acid or alkaline urine) is calcium oxalate or calcium carbonate stones.
Many stones are mixed types.
Acid urine: uric acid, cystine, xanthine
Alkaline urine (order of frequency): calcium, magnesium, ammonium phosphates

Special Features

1. Usually occur in 3rd and 4th decade, rare in children and over age 50
2. Dangerous because they produce obstruction and infection
3. Small stones, < 0.5 cm., pass into ureter. Larger stones remain in renal pelvis; may become staghorn calculi

Prophylaxis

Vitamin A
Beer

DIVERTICULA

Urinary Bladder

1. Congenital, with muscle in the wall
2. Acquired, without muscle in the wall
   a. Secondary to increased pressure
   b. Much more common than congenital
   c. Most common in males with BPH
   d. They are present in 10% to 15% of patients over 50 at autopsy

Urethra

1. Congenital urethral valves with vesical neck obstruction (RARE). Causes: hypospadias, hydronephrosis, infection. Symptoms: large residual volume of urine and straining to void
2. Urethrorectal fistula often accompanies IMPERFORATE ANUS
3. Diverticulum of urethra RARE, almost exclusively in females

INFECTIONS

Urinary tract obstruction is the primary cause

Ureteritis and Cystitis Cystica

a. *USUALLY* associated with long-standing GU infections
b. Infolding of mucosa and metaplasia; von Brunn crypts form cysts with mucin plugs
c. Berry-like projections along ureter; larger in bladder than in ureter

Encrusted Ureteritis or Cystitis

a. Necrotic mucosa with encrustation
b. Usually associated with *urea-splitting organisms: Proteus vulgaris,* staph and *E. coli*
Symptoms: gravel and high pH of urine

Gonococcal Ureteritis (Specific)

Gram-negative, intracellular diplococcus of Neisser

Nonspecific Ureteritis

a. More than one organism USUALLY found
b. USUALLY associated with prostatitis

Tuberculosis of Urinary Tract

a. Almost always secondary to TB of kidney
b. May involve mucosa or wall

Honeymoon Cystitis

Any organism

INFLAMMATIONS

SPECIAL TYPES

Hunner Ulcer (Chronic Interstitial Cystitis)

1. Almost always in females
2. Intramural fibrosis (scar) and inflammation with decreased blood supply, so get ulcer, bleeding with overdistention
3. Symptoms: marked frequency, day and night (small capacity), with terminal burning

Radiation Cystitis

1. MOST common with treated carcinoma of cervix
2. Acute: erythema, edema, granulation tissue with round cells, necrosis if severe
3. Chronic: fibrosis, round cells, endarteritis (SCAR)

Malakoplakia (Soft Plaque; RARE)

1. Giant cells with basophilic inclusion bodies (Michaelis-Gutman bodies) which are often *iron-positive* and *calcium-positive;* similar to Schaumann bodies in sarcoid
2. Macrophages, lymphocytes, and plasma cells
3. Michaelis-Gutman bodies are also called calcospherites

TUMORS

Ureter

1. Ureter carcinoma rare, hematuria most common presenting sign
2. Pathology:
   Papillary: similar to papillary bladder carcinoma
   Solid (nonpapillary): transitional or squamous cell carcinoma
3. Prognosis: poor, symptoms come late

Urethra

1. Carcinoma rare
2. MOST common type in males is squamous (epidermoid) carcinoma
3. In females USUALLY is extension of cervical carcinoma

CARCINOMAS

Urinary Bladder

Etiology	Key words: Analine dye workers (beta naphthalene), schistosomiasis in Egypt, and tobacco use
Symptoms	Painless hematuria (75% present with painless hematuria)
Pathology	1. 90% papillary (low-grade tumors)
	2. 10% sessile (higher grade tumors)
Micro	1. 90% transitional cell carcinoma
	2. 10% squamous cell carcinoma, especially with schistosomiasis
	3. 1%–2% adenocarcinoma, usually at dome with extrophy of bladder
Prognosis	Based on extension, NOT on microscopic appearance (Broder's classification)

Staging: Modified Jewett's Classification

Stage	Location	5-Year Survival
0	Carcinoma in situ	Nearly 100%
A	Submucosa only	90%
B_1	Superficial muscle	80%
B_2	Deep muscle	26%
C	Through muscle	8%
D	Infiltration into adjacent organs	0–10%

Note

Transitional cell carcinoma may also occur in ureters, renal pelvis, and oral cavity
Cause of death: (1) ureteral obstruction with uremia; (2) said not to cause widespread metastasis, but can occasionally

Treatment

1. Papillary
   Usually resected by TUR, fulguration, and observe
2. Sessile
   a. Segmental resection
   b. Cystectomy with
      1) ileal drainage pouch, urinary sepsis (29%)
      2) ureterosigmoidostomy
         a) hyperchloremic acidosis (49%)
         b) urinary sepsis (44%)
      3) Can also give supervoltage radiation

SOME OTHER TUMORS

SARCOMA BOTRYOIDES

Polypoid rhabdomyosarcoma, usually in vagina or uterus of children, but can arise from bladder

Micro

Myxomatous stroma with striated muscle (probably a mixed mesodermal tumor or a variant of rhabdomyosarcoma)

NEWER CONCEPTS

1. So far urinary bladder is the only place where an asymmetric unit membrane (AUM) has been found
2. AUM of urinary bladder has 5 layers (3 electron-dense, 2 electron-lucent); thickest portion of AUM is faced toward lumen and vesicles of bladder cells, which become part of mucosal surface in expanded bladder
3. AUM assembled in and by Golgi apparatus, supranuclearly in intermediate cells of bladder epithelium, no AUM in basal cells
4. AUM probably what keeps urine from leaking from bladder
5. Since bladder does not have any mucosal folds, villi or microvilli-like intestine, presence of deep AUM-lined vesicles connected with surface in contracted bladder allow bladder epithelial cells to present a uniform AUM-lined surface to urine-containing lumen, even in expanded state
6. Source of thickened "surface coat" on the AUM is disputed; may be from substances in urine, or may be added by epithelial cells only when vesicles are in contact with the luminal surface
7. On EM, the AUM is *consistently associated* with lysosomes, which probably store useless or damaged AUM

23 Male Genitals

	Penis
Lesions	*Key Words*

Significant Benign

Phimosis — Definition: orifice of prepuce too small to permit retraction of foreskin

Paraphimosis — Definition: retracted foreskin that cannot be replaced

Balanitis — Nonspecific (usually bacterial) infection of glans and prepuce with edema, ulceration, and inflammation

Peyronie's disease, penile fibromatosis, cavernositis
1. Fibromatosis fasciitis of penis shaft, most commonly superior but may be lateral
2. Peak occurrence in 4th decade
3. Frequently associated with Dupuytren's contracture; etiology unknown
4. Key symptoms: pain on erection and displacement toward fibrosis with erection
5. Micro: identical with keloid

Benign Tumors

Condyloma acuminatum
1. A benign, villous, papillary growth of unknown etiology thought by some to be sexually transmitted
2. On the penis, the most common location is the coronal sulcus
3. Micro: branching, villous, papillary connective tissue stroma with hyperplastic, hyperkeratotic, acanthotic epithelium

Giant condyloma (Buschke-Lowenstein tumor)
1. Giant (large) benign, may appear multifocal
2. May be locally invasive and destructive, no metastases
3. Treated with local radical excision

Premalignant

Erythroplasia of Queyrat
1. Limited to glans penis; red plaques
2. Epithelial dysplasia, hyperplasia, and hyperkeratosis
3. Present years before cancer

Bowen's disease
1. Carcinoma in situ on shaft of penis; 8% become invasive carcinoma
2. Corps rond

Leukoplakia — White plaque

(Continued on overleaf)

135

Penis *(continued)*

Lesions	Key Words

Malignant
  Squamous cell carcinoma
	1. Most common malignant tumor of penis
	2. Etiology
	    a. Smegma (circumcision protects)
	    b. Commonly associated with chronic irritation, phimosis, etc.
	    c. Most common in area of glans penis
	    d. 50% 5-year survival

PROSTATE

BENIGN PROSTATIC HYPERTROPHY (BPH)

Etiology

Unknown, (?) hormonal imbalance

Clinical

1. Frequency, hesitancy, dribbling, nocturia (most common cause of urinary obstruction in postpubertal males)
2. Very common after age 50

Gross

Lateral lobes enlarged, firm, but NOT stony hard
Prostate may weigh up to 100 grams

Micro

Fibromuscular stromal hypertrophy and hyperplasia with glandular hyperplasia and dilatation; corpora amylacea frequently seen

Notes

1. No elevation of acid phosphatase
2. May get hydroureter and hydronephrosis as complications
3. Treatment: usually transurethral resection without orchiectomy

ADENOCARCINOMA

General Statements

1. Very common cancer in old men
2. Rarely occurs in areas of BPH
3. Areas of infarction commonly mistaken microscopically for carcinoma of prostate
4. 90% occur in posterior lobe

Etiology

Hormonal imbalance (?)

Clinical

1. Symptoms: urethral obstruction late, "stony" hard on rectal exam
2. Bone pain with metastases
3. Produces osteoblastic lesions (elevated alkaline phosphatase)

4. Acid phosphatase (tartrate-sensitive) elevated with extension beyond capsule
5. Acid phosphatase (tartrate-sensitive) does *not* elevate without extension beyond capsule
6. Do 5' nucleotidase, leucine amino peptidase, or gamma glutamyl transpeptidase to differentiate bone from liver alkaline phosphatase

Pathology

	Occult (Tumor confined to gland)	Aggressive (Tumor extending beyond capsule)
Incidence	Skid Row series: 60% of males over 70 years Most series: 29% over 70	3rd most common cause of cancer deaths in males
Gross	Firm, yellow-white posterior lobe	Yellow, crablike, firm lesions, posterior lobe; stony hard
Micro	Carcinoma in gland Perineural lymphatic invasion best criteria	Spread beyond gland Can go to brain without invading internal organs (via Bateson's plexus)
Therapy	TUR and orchectomy is as good as any, without complications of radical surgery Mortality higher with estrogen than without, especially in 1st year	(Same as for occult)
Course	Usually long	Protracted
5-Year survival	Over 70%	33%
Note	Prognosis is roughly correlated with the stage of the disease, (e.g., extension) and less well correlated with grading (e.g., Broder's classification). There are several staging systems without universal agreement among experts in the area.	

TESTES

CRYPTORCHIDISM

Etiology and Pathogenesis

1. Lack of chorionic gonadotropin hormone (2%)
2. Mechanical—ring too small, short cord, etc. (98%)

Incidence

1. Most common congenital anomaly of testis
2. 1 of 25 males under 14 years; 1 in 250 males over 21 years
3. 20% bilateral
4. 70%–100% accompanied by inguinal hernia

Symptoms

NONE; sterility if bilateral

Pathology

Location: 60% inguinal, 14% intraabdominal, 26% outer inguinal ring
Micro: Until puberty, not different from undescended; after puberty, progressive atrophy, thickened BM of tubules, loss of spermatogenesis, few Sertoli cells persist, interstitial fibrosis and hyperplasia of Leydig cells

Special Features

1. Chorionic gonadotropin; 10%–20% descend with it; do orchiopexy after puberty if hormone does not work
2. Most serious complication is increased incidence of carcinoma, seminoma most common; 10% of cryptorchids become cancerous; 0.001% of normally located testes become cancerous

Tunica Diseases

	Hydrocele	Spermatocele	Hematocele
Etiology	1. Serous fluid (between visceral and parietal layers of tunica vaginalis) 2. Most common cause of scrotal swelling in U.S.A. 3. 90% occur over 21 years of age 4. Most commonly associated with inflammation of epididymis	Trauma or inflammation, blocking of epididymis and spermatic ducts	1. Absence (?) of gubernaculum testis 2. Uncommon 3. Most commonly associated with torsion of spermatic cord due to trauma
Clinical	Key word: TRANSILLUMINATION	Dilated epididymis filled with spermatoza	Hemorrhage
Pathology	Atrophic testes, fluid and sac	Testicular atrophy	Hemosiderosis, fibrous atrophy
Usual amounts of fluid	100–300 cc., with trauma can get hydrohematocele	5–20 cc.	100 cc.

SPERMATIC GRANULOMA

Most frequently seen as a complication of vas ligation; positive FANA test with anti-DNA antibodies; (?) autoimmune disease

Germinal Neoplasms of the Testes

Group	I	II	III	IV	V
	Pure Seminoma	Embryonal Carcinoma Pure or with Seminoma	Teratoma (Pure or with Seminoma)	Teratocarcinoma with Embryonal Cell Carcinoma or Choriocarcinoma with or Without Seminoma	Choriocarcinoma
Etiology	Undescended testes Unknown	(?)	Germinal cell nests	(?)	(?)
Radiation	Very sensitive	Not sensitive	Slightly sensitive	Not sensitive	Not sensitive
Symptoms	Usually not painful	90% HAVE ENLARGEMENT OF TESTES — 50% HAVE PAIN (AN UNFAVORABLE PROGNOSTIC SIGN)			
Relative percentage of malignant testicular tumors	38	20	8	31	1
Age group	ALL ARE HIGHEST IN 25–40-YEAR-OLD GROUP				
Gross	Large, soft, pale, homogenous	Usually not large, gray-white, mottled, hemorrhagic	Variable size, commonly focal cysts, not homogenous	Variable size, less cystic than teratoma	Only slight enlargement of testis
Micro	Uniform, large polygonal cells with "ground-glass" cytoplasm. Focal granulomas may be seen. Lymphoid stroma	Anaplastic cells. Epithelial-lined clefts. No lymphoid stroma	Adult-looking, variable pattern, any germ layer—cartilage, epithelium, etc.	Malignant-looking pattern with any germ layer present	1. Cytotrophoblasts 2. Syncytiotrophoblasts 3. Villus-like structures (no true villi)
Chorionic gonadotropin secreted	Very uncommon	About 33%	About 25%	Up to 25%	80%–90%
5-Year survival and Rx	89% Orchiectomy, radiation of periaortic nodes	25% Orchiectomy, retroperitoneal node dissection, radiation if seminoma present	68% Orchiectomy with retroperitoneal node dissection, radiation if seminoma present	36% Orchiectomy, radiation if seminoma present	0 Orchiectomy Methotrexate does not cure

Nongerminal Tumors of the Testes

	Adenomatoid Tumor	Sertoli Cell Tumor	Interstitial Cell Tumor
Incidence	Rare	Very rare (PURE Sertoli cell tumor)	Rare, most common in the middle adult life
Histogenesis	Form of mesothelioma	Sertoli cells	Leydig cell component same as arrhenoblastoma in females
Clinical	Also seen in female genital tract (usually fallopian tubes)	Feminization, gynecomastia	Prepubertal: precocious puberty Postpubertal: often no symptoms Old age: "Daddy blooms again"
Pathology			
Gross	Small, gray tumor, usually in superior pole of testes	Small, homogenous	Small (1–2 cm.), yellow-brown
Micro	Cords, nests, glands and stroma	Hyperplastic Sertoli cells, loss of spermatogenic elements	Nests and sheets of hyperplastic Leydig cells with eosinophilic granular cytoplasm, crystalloids of Reinke in cytoplasm, tubular atrophy
Special features	1. Benign, *NO* malignant potential 2. Commonly mistaken for adenocarcinoma	1. Feminization 2. Usually mixed with Leydig cells, also seen in ovary as Sertoli-Leydig tumor	1. 10% malignant 2. Some produce feminization, Sertoli-Leydig tumor

Note: About 2/3 of embryonal cell carcinomas have increased serum alpha fetoprotein (AFP); uncommonly AFP may be elevated in other tumors

24 Vulva, Vagina and Cervix

VULVAR CARCINOMA

CLINICAL

Usually seen in over-age-60 group
Commonly associated with leukoplakia and kraurosis
Previous granulomatous disease, 40%
3rd most common female genital cancer after cervix and ovary

PATHOLOGICAL

Gross

Usually focal, maplike, white areas, often with ulceration and eczematoid appearance
May occur in condylomata

Micro

Usually well-differentiated squamous cell carcinomas
Basal cell tumors commonly associated with granulomatous disease

Therapy

Radical vulvectomy with node dissection

Prognosis

30%–40% overall 5-year survival
Approximately 60% show distant metastases by time of diagnosis
Metastasis correlates better with size and duration of tumor than with micro appearance

CARCINOMA IN SITU

CLINICAL

Usually a focal, white lesion, occasionally with eczematoid appearance (common in older age group)

PATHOLOGICAL

Gross

Usually a focal, white area, with or without ulcerations or reddened background

Micro

Acanthosis, hyperkeratosis, dyskeratosis, anaplastic appearing cells; atypical maturation with *complete* loss of normal stratification and absence of superficial cells, Bowenoid changes, "corps ronds", frequently seen

Therapy

Simple vulvectomy

Prognosis

Excellent

BARTHOLIN GLAND (VULVOVAGINAL) CYST

Usually results from obstruction or following absorption of abscesses
Gonorrhea or trichomonas most commonly precede

Key Features

	Acute Stage	Chronic Stage
Gross	Swollen, edematous labia majora, usually unilateral Often purulent with pus from duct orifice	Enlarged, hard gland readily felt Cysts develop due to occlusion of ducts
Micro	Shows heavy infiltration of PMN leukocytes, edema, epithelial degeneration, desquamation	Shows transitional to flattened epithelium or absence due to pressure atrophy, or lined by chronic inflammatory or granulomatous tissue

LEUKOPLAKIA

What is it?

Schwimmer (1877): Precancerous lesion of the tongue
Breisky (1885): Atrophic, whitish, constrictive; change similar to kraurosis
Taussig (1929): Recognized hypertrophic and atrophic forms, believed malignant potential was equal in both forms; recognized 3 stages progressing from hypertrophic to atrophic
Bonney (1938): Recognized it as an inflammatory condition with atrophic and hypertrophic forms; thought hypertrophic form preceded atrophic form; though only hypertrophic form had malignant potential

PRESENT CONCEPTS

Clinical

Focal, white, premalignant lesion, often associated with kraurosis and pruritus vulvae

TO THE PATHOLOGIST

Gross

Circumscribed white lesion having:
1. Erythema, edema, excoriations
2. Thickened, whitened vulvar folds
3. Cracking, superficial ulceration, and bluish-white skin

Micro

Hyperkeratosis, acanthosis with bizarre anaplasticoid immature cells at basal rete pegs; transitional or basal cell tumor commonly seen in areas preceded by granulomatous lesions

PATHOLOGICAL "GRADING"

Grade I—Hyperplastic Vulvitis

Commonly associated with chronic dermatitis, rarely malignant
Micro: Mild hyperkeratosis; regular—without distortion—acanthotic rete pegs; few inflammatory cells
Therapy: Control patient's symptoms, observe

Grade II—True Leukoplakia

Will become cancer in 25%–66%
Micro: Marked hyperkeratosis, acanthosis, atypical maturation deep at rete pegs, dyskeratosis, collagenation and marked inflammatory cell infiltrate common, NO invasion of dermis
Therapy: Simple vulvectomy
Note Carcinoma can develop without dramatic aberrations, especially in areas with previous granulomatous disease

Lichen Sclerosus et Atrophicus

	Hypertrophic	*Atrophic*
Clinical	Focal, benign white or bluish lesion of the vulva; pruritus vulvae common (often both types are mixed in same patient)	
Pathological		
Gross	Focal, white cracked skin	Focal, bluish-white skin
Micro	Hyperkeratoses, acanthoses, and dipping down of rete pegs; some chronic inflammatory cell infiltrate in upper dermis; no anaplasticoid proliferation at rete peg tips; no dyskeratoses	Thin keratin layer, thin epidermis, loss of rete pegs, collagenation at dermis, decreased numbers of chronic inflammatory cells
Note	—————— Malignancy may develop in 2%–3% of cases ——————	
Therapy	—————— Biopsy, control symptoms, observe patient ——————	

KRAUROSIS

Definition

1. Clinical term for shrinkage and loss of vulvar structures
2. Often associated with whitish discoloration and pruritus vulvae
3. Microscopically identical with lichen sclerosus et atrophicus; may have appearance of leukoplakia grossly
4. This diagnosis cannot be made with microscope

Therapy

Control symptoms and biopsy suspicious lesions (simple vulvectomy for intractable pruritus)

BENIGN TUMORS

HYDRADENOMA PAPILLIFERUM

Skin tumor, MOST often on vulva, found in axilla also; *often confused with carcinoma*

Micro

Adenomatous pattern with many tubular ducts, single/double layer of nonciliated columnar cells with clear cytoplasm, beneath which is a layer of flattened myoepithelial cells

URETHRAL CARBUNCLE

Etiology

From chronically infected urethral mucosa

Signs and Symptoms

Atrophy of vaginal mucosa, often no presenting symptoms

Gross

Reddened, polypoid lesion, usually on posterior portion of meatus

Micro

Three forms described:
Papillomatous: Edema, transitional stratified squamous epithelium
Angiomatous: Many small vessels, edema, epithelium may be absent
Granulomatous: Inflammatory cells, edema, epithelium may be absent

GONORRHEAL VULVOVAGINITIS

Etiology

In infants & children: direct contact with pus-containing *Neisseria gonorrhoeae*
In sexually mature females: sexual contact with *N. gonorrhoeae* primarily in glands associated with vulva/urethra

Signs and Symptoms

In children: violent inflammatory reaction, vulva/vagina fiery red, swollen

In adult females: purulent exudate

Micro

In children: thin, atrophic epithelial layer of cells and ulceration; subepithelial connective tissue infiltrated with round and plasma cells
In adult females: round cell infiltrate in connective tissue

Special Features

1. Newborn females resistant because of thick vaginal epithelium due to mother's HORMONES
2. From 6 months to puberty females very susceptible because of low, thin epithelium due to NO hormonal stimulation

Malignant Tumors of the Vagina

	Carcinoma	*Sarcoma Botryoides*
Origin, onset and course	Most are squamous cell; Uncommon to rare, posterior wall, upper half most often, Any age, most often late childbearing period High incidence of vaginal adenosis and adenocarcinoma in teenage girls whose mothers were treated with diethylstilbestrol while girls were in utero	Rare, usually in upper vagina and cervix, most common in infants and young children, from totipotential mesenchymal cells, rapid growth and death, USUALLY within a year; metastasizes locally and distantly, bloody discharge frequent
Gross	Forms a. Papillary b. Noduloulcerative c. Infiltrating All forms ulcerate and indurate	*Grapelike masses* of blue-white tissue; in infant, this is almost pathognomonic
Micro	*Primary* Epidermoid type (95%) Adenocarcinoma (5%) Melanoma (rare) *Metastatic* Usually more common than primary from cervix, ovary, stomach	Mesenchymatous pattern reminiscent of embryonal form of rhabdomyosarcoma
Special features	Primary carcinoma of vagina is rare, usually extends from cervix or vulva or is metastatic	1. Also may arise in bladder 2. May be a mixed mesodermal tumor

CERVIX

BENIGN LESIONS

Chronic Cervicitis

1. The MOST common lesion of the adult cervix; present in nearly 100% of postpubertal females
2. Frequently have cysts called *nabothian cysts;* frequently multiple and originate from occluded orifices of cervical glands by mucin or edema
3. Doubtful relationship to cancer if severe

Malignant and Premalignant Lesions of the Cervix

	Basal Cell Dysplasia (Hyperplasia) (BCH)	*Carcinoma in Situ BCH Class, Grade 4/Class IV*	*Carcinoma*
Etiology	Unknown, severe chronic cervicitis most common	SEX—(?) HSV-2	SEX, smegma—HSV-2 antibodies, herpes genitalis (80%)
Signs and symptoms	Usually no symptoms, bleeding rare, peak age is 30–35 years	Usually no symptoms, vaginal bleeding rare, peak age 35 years	Vaginal discharge, contact bleeding, peak age 45 years
Gross	Cervix reddened, congested, edematous Schiller's iodine test = Gram's iodine stains normal cervix mahogany brown, eroded areas remain unstained, *no glycogen*	Eroded cervix, bleeds easily and usually enlarged, scars frequently seen, discharge	Ulceration or induration with erosion of ulcer margins, may be fungating growth
Micro	Basal cell hyperplasia (dysplasia), atypical metaplasia, basal cells extending beyond basal quarter of epithelium	Hyperchromatic atypical basal cells extend throughout ENTIRE thickness of epithelium, but no tumor below BM and no glycogen on surface Need PAS stain to make positive diagnosis in some cases	1. 95% squamous cell Ca 2. 5% adenocarcinomas 3. Most are low-grade tumors with keratin pearls 4. Tumor must extend below basement membrane 5. May need PAS stain to confirm in early cases
Prognosis and classification	1. 5-year survival 100% 2. 25% untreated cases of 3/III develop into carcinoma in situ	Carcinoma of cervix Stage 0, nearly 100% 5-year survival	

Broder's Classification

Grade (Broders's)	Class	Basal Cell Thickness	Prognosis
1	I	25%	Normal
2	II	50%	Benign
3	III	75%	25% become Ca
4	IV	100%	Carcinoma in situ

MODIFIED LEAGUE OF NATIONS CLASSIFICATION FOR CARCINOMA OF THE CERVIX (LON)

Stage 0 (Carcinoma in situ)

Carcinoma confined to the intraepithelial area, not extending below BM

Stage I

Carcinoma strictly confined to cervix
85% 5-year survival

Stage II

Carcinoma extends beyond cervix but has not reached pelvic wall; entire broad ligament on one or both sides may be involved; carcinoma involves the vagina but not lower third; carcinoma extends into endometrial cavity from endocervix
75% 5-year survival

Stage III

Carcinoma has reached pelvic wall; on rectal examination, no cancer-free space found between tumor and pelvic wall; carcinoma involves lower third of vagina
50% 5-year survival

Stage IV

Carcinoma has invaded adjacent viscera, involving bladder, rectum, or both; vesicovaginal or rectovaginal fistulas may be present
10% 5-year survival

POLYPS

Mucous (Endocervical)

Most common, hyperplastic, often pedunculated, rarely sessile, stroma edematous and lined with columnar epithelium—usually singular

Squamous (Ectocervical)

Less common, often sessile and in area of external os, usually symptomless, contact bleeding most common symptom

Treatment

1. Infection often a cause of leukorrhea; include base when excising
2. DO NOT excise in office (may cause fatal hemorrhage)
3. Rx: excision, include base when excising

25 Corpus Uteri and Pregnancy

ENDOMETRIUM

Menstrual Cycle

Menstruation	Proliferative	Secretory	Premenstrual
Days			
1–4	5–14 (ovulation)	14–26	22–28
Hormones			
Progesterone decreased	FSH increases Estrogen formed Endometrium regenerates	Starts at time of ovulation Progesterone matures stroma	Starts 8–10 days after ovulation, continues to Day 1 of menses Progesterone decreases
Glands			
Endometrial glands necrose and slough due to prior constriction of coiled arteries	1. Glands lengthen 2. Cells multiply and become tall, columnar 3. Pseudostratification of nuclei of glands 4. Gland mitosis seen	1. *Secretory:* vacuoles at base of cells below nuclei; *first* (histological) evidence of ovulation 2. Glands dilate and become tortuous (vacuoles migrate to exposed ends of cells; 3–8 mm. of thick mucosa) 3. Glands secrete mucus in lumina	1. Tortuosity and size of glands greatly increase 2. Much glycogen in glands
Stromata			
Thin, edematous, vascular, many polys	Dense, compact, nonvacuolated cells	1. Large, plump, vacuolated cells 2. Edematous toward end 3. Increased inflammatory cells toward end	1. Cells become large, polyhedral and pale staining 2. Edema, vascularity increases 3. Vessels become tortuous 4. Many polys

Endometriosis

	Direct (Adenomyosis; Interna)	Indirect (Chocolate Cysts; Externa)
Etiology	(?), trauma may separate muscle bundles	*Sampson theory (1921):* menstrual regurgitation *Objections:* cannot explain extracoelomic endometriosis *Coelomic metaplasia theory*
Signs and symptoms	1. Menorrhagia 2. *Colicky dysmenorrhea*—due to swelling under tension	1. Usually in white patients 30–40 years old 2. May be symptomless 3. Dysmenorrhea with referred pain may occur
Location	In or on myometrium	Order of frequency: 1. Ovary, (chocolate cysts) 2. Uterosacral ligaments 3. Rectovaginal septum 4. Round ligaments, also umbilicus, (Cullen's sign, blue nodules), laparotomy scars, appendix, intestines, and elsewhere
Gross	Uterus slightly to moderately enlarged with uncircumscribed, whorled appearance (red-colored areas)	*Young:* pinpoint and larger bluish or reddish brown, spongy (chocolate) cysts *Old:* scar, simulates cancer with adhesions
Micro	1. Endometrial islands within muscular layer 2. Endometrial tissue should be at least 1 HPF below basal endometrium 3. *NO* cyclic changes, sequestered or unripe (?)	1. Endometrial tissue (glands and stroma in or on tissue or organ involved) 2. Later, hemosiderin pigment, fibrosis scar 3. Undergoes *cyclic changes* while the lesion is young
Special features	Rarely gives rise to malignancy	1. Malignancy rare 2. Commonly mistaken (clinically and grossly) for carcinoma

Endometritis

	Acute	Chronic
Etiology	Almost exclusively postpartum disease, group-A beta-hemolytic streptococcus most common organism, gonococcus rarely causes it	Usually with PID secondary to gonococcus or from tuberculosis salpingitis, a disputed entity except for tuberculosis
Signs and symptoms (gross and micro)	Endometrium swollen, hyperemic, edematous, leukocytic (PMN) infiltrate, bleeding with foul discharge	Inflammatory infiltration of endometrium, mostly composed of *plasma cells* and few mononuclear cells
Special features	Uncommon because endometrium is resistant to infection and self-cleaning	Giant cells suggest acid-fast infection, granulomata, foreign bodies

Hyperplasia of Endometrium

	"Swiss Cheese" Hyperplasia	Adenomatous (Atypical) Hyperplasia
Etiology	Excess estrogenic stimulation via (1) follicle persistence (2) granulosa theca cell tumors of ovary (3) adrenocortical hormones	
Signs and symptoms	————————————— Bleeding after menopause —————————————	
Gross	Varies; but endometrium is *greatly overgrown,* curettage may yield much *polyploid* tissue; necrosis and friability usually absent	
Micro	Increase in epithelial and stromal elements Large glands usually lined with layer of epithelium *Much* variation in size of cystic glands, large and small are seen	Increase in "epithelial glands" and stromal elements Pseudostratification of gland epithelium, often back-to-back glands, resembles adenocarcinoma *Little variation* in size of glands
Special features	NOT precancerous Uterine bleeding May be associated with estrogen-secreting tumor	Considered precancerous; up to 75% develop into carcinoma Uterine bleeding May be associated with estrogen-secreting tumor "Nicht karzinoma, besser heraus"

"The Pill" and the Endometrium

Depending on the type and ratio of estrogen/progesterone-like drugs taken, different endometrial effects are produced. High estrogen will produce excess glandular proliferation. Progesterone generally produces stromal hyperplasia and "metaplasia" to a deciduoid type of stroma reminiscent of pregnancy. The main problem of the pill for the pathologist is mistaking its effects for tumorous conditions, including pregnancy.

Polyps of Endometrium

	Placental	Adenomatous
Etiology	*True:* rare *Pseudo:* retained placenta	Menopausal
Signs and symptoms	Bleeding, enlarged uterus focally	Continuous or intermittent bleeding, soft uterus
Special considerations	Grossly soft, friable, and hemorrhagic, may resemble adenocarcinoma	
	Old villi and decidua render it indistinguishable from incomplete abortion *"Arias-stella"* phenomenon in endometrium may resemble adenocarcinoma on micro	Micro shows closely packed glands, may resemble adenocarcinoma or hyperplasia Carcinomatous changes often occur Some remain unripe, some cycle with rest of endometrium

MALIGNANT ENDOMETRIAL TUMORS

ADENOCARCINOMA

Etiology

1. Hormonal (estrogen/progesterone imbalance)
2. Associated conditions: hyperestrinism (external or internal), obesity, hypertension, diabetes, nulliparity, thyroid disease, breast carcinoma
3. Poor obstetrical care

Signs and Symptoms

1. Menorrhagia
2. Metrorrhagia

Gross

Diffuse: friable, bulky and extensive
Circumscribed: focal polypoid mass, usually on a pedicle or polyp

Micro

Hyperplastic glands, back-to-back, and disorderly

Special Features

1. Adenoacanthoma 10%, (squamous metaplasia), occuring with adenocarcinoma of the endometrium, no change in prognosis
2. Usually in 50–60 age group, 10 years later than cervical Ca
3. Increasing in relative ratio to Ca of cervix

Prognosis

Criteria:

Stage 0: histology suspicious for carcinoma in situ, 100% curable
Stage 1: carcinoma confined to corpus, 70–90% curable
Stage 2: carcinoma involves corpus and cervix, 50% curable

Stage 3: carcinoma extends outside uterus, but not outside true pelvis, 25% curable
Stage 4a: carcinoma involves *mucosa* of bladder or rectum, 0% curable
Stage 4b: any stage as above, plus nodal spread and metastasis outside pelvis, 0% curable

Overall 5-year survival with treatment (except Stage 4):

Radiation and surgery survival (60%)
Irradiation alone (33%)
Surgery alone (50%)

UTERUS

Leiomyomata (Fibroid, Myoma, Fibromyoma)

Etiology	Heredity (?), Black race more common, ovarian hormones (?) (bigger in pregnancy and shrink postmenopausally)
Signs and symptoms	Pressure lower pelvis, infertility, abortion, dystocia
Gross	Vary from microscopic growths to the size of an orange (record size is over 100 pounds) All are pseudoencapsulated and have whorled cut surface

Location	*Intramural*	*Subserosal*	*Submucous*
	Nodular, in wall only	Often pedicled, occasionally becomes parasitic, projects from serous surface	Protrudes into uterus

Micro	1. Histogenesis from smooth muscle, monoclonal by G6PD assay 2. Whorled bundles of elevated cells running in all directions 3. A few mast cells may be seen

Secondary Changes (Degeneration) of Uterine Myoma

1. Hyaline degeneration most common
2. Cystic degeneration: irregular cavities filled with gelatinous material
3. Calcification: circulatory impairment; "womb stone"; rare in submucous myomas
4. Infection/suppuration—in submucous types most often
5. Necrosis occurs in any type of myoma due to altered blood supply; red degeneration-special variation of necrosis, in pregnancy usually
6. Fatty changes uncommon; sequel to hyaline degeneration or necrosis
7. Sarcomatous degeneration occurs in less than 1% of myomata

PLACENTA

NORMAL DATA

Hormones

Syncytiotrophoblast is origin of all placental hormones, HCG, chroionic growth hormone, lactogen, estrogen and progesterone

Gross

Term placenta: 450–500 g. normal weight, cotyledons (12–20) on maternal surface

Micro

Fetal blood vessels comprise 1/3–2/3 of villi at term

Hofbauer cells: large mononuclear phagocytes; *Cytotrophoblast:* has mitotic figures; *Syncytium:* has no mitotic figures, contains much ER, Golgi, mitochondria, secretory droplets, lipid granules and plasma membranes

Villi composed of
1. Connective tissue
2. Fetal vessels
3. Hofbauer cells
4. Chorionic epithelium, composed of
   a. Cytotrophoblast (Langhans' cells), inner layer, may have mitotic figures, precursor cell
   b. Syncytiotrophoblast (outer layer): contains much ER, Golgi, secretory droplets and vacuoles, makes ALL placental hormones, these nuclei form syncytial knots

Common Benign Diseases of Placenta

	Eclampsia	Syphilis	Erythroblastosis Fetalis (Hemolytic Disease of Newborn -HDN)
Etiology	Toxemia (?)	*Treponema pallidum*	Rh or other incompatibility between mother and fetus, usually Rh (D)
Signs and symptoms	A symptom complex of hypertension, proteinuria, edema, convulsions	Syphilis in mother	Death of fetus in 3rd trimester
Gross	Placenta: small, fibrotic, with frequent infarcts (premature aging)	Enlarged placenta (up to 2000 gm. at term)	Edematous, large, pale placenta up to 2000 gm. at term
Micro	1. Loss of syncytium (naked villi) 2. Increased syncytial knots 3. Increased intervillous thrombosis 4. Hyaline degeneration of villi and fetal vessel walls	1. Bulbous swelling and fibrosis of villi 2. Obliterative endarteritis 3. Perivascular plasma cells 4. Atrophy of villi	1. Relative immaturity 2. Edema early 3. Excess Hofbauer cells 4. Enlarged clubbed villi 5. Persistent Langhans' cells 6. Atrophy late
Special features	1. Toxemia, often followed by shock 2. Thromboses in vessels of liver and kidneys, brain, and pituitary of mother 3. Focal peripheral lobular necrosis in maternal liver also seen	Very rare now Treponema can only cross the placenta after 5th month of pregnancy	1. Occurs in 1:200 births 2. RHO-GAM, (IgG) passive immunity, now protects 3. RHO-GAM must be given *before* anti-Rh(D) titer develops

Malignant Diseases of Placenta

	Hydatidiform Mole (Neoplastic ?)	Chorioadenoma Destruens (Invasive Hydatidiform Mole)	Choriocarcinoma Chorionepithelioma
Etiology	1. Inadequate diet in Far East, Mexico (1:200 to 1:350 pregnancies) 2. Low HCG in Chinese–(1:100 pregnancies) 3. In U.S.A., 1:2500 pregnancies	Trophoblastic proliferation, unknown (?) Blighted ovum	1:40,000 pregnancies in U.S.A. (?) 50% from previous hydatidiform mole 25% from previous abortion 22% from normal pregnancies
Signs and symptoms	Enlarged uterus, no pain	Enlarged uterus, bleeding due to vascular invasion (hemoperitoneum or vaginal bleeding)	Enlarged uterus, uterine bleeding
Gross	*Grapelike particles,* no fetus, "blighted ovum"	Tumor invading uterine wall	Tumor associated with hemorrhage, coagulation necrosis
Micro	1. Well-preserved villous pattern 2. Hydropic degeneration of villi 3. Piling trophoblastic cells 4. No tendency to penetrate stroma 5. No destructive invasion of uterine tissues	1. Proliferated syncytial + cytotrophoblast 2. Highly vascular tumor invades locally 3. Villi usually present	1. Chorionic villi *absent* 2. Clusters of cytotrophoblasts, streams of large syncytial cells 3. *Much hemorrhage*
Special	1. Trophoblasts rarely may be in mother's lungs with spontaneous lysis after delivery 2. Not malignant, 81% follow a benign course 3. Follow with HCG levels, usually high 4. 2.5% become choriocarcinoma 5. 16% become chorioadenoma destruens	1. Local invasive mole without metastases 2. Increased levels of HCG 3. Differentiate from choriocarcinoma by lack of viable metastases, biologic behavior, and villi	1. Methotrexate cures 2. Follow therapy with HCG levels 3. U.S.A.: 1 in 40 hydatidiform moles; becomes choriocarcinoma 4. U.S.A.: 1 in 160,000 NORMAL pregnancies becomes choriocarcinoma

26 Ovaries and Tubes

Miscellaneous Diseases of the Ovaries

	Stein-Leventhal Syndrome	Follicle Cysts	Lutein Cysts
Etiology	Thick capsule, enzyme block (?) Chromosomal defect (?)	Unruptured graafian follicles	Excess progesterone (?)
Signs and symptoms	Occurs in late teens, early 20's 1. Obesity 2. Hirsutism 3. Menstrual irregularity 4. Amenorrhea 5. Reduced fertility to sterility	Hemorrhage into cysts gives inflammatory symptoms	Unilateral pain
Gross	1. Bilateral large white ovaries with cortical-stromal fibrosis 2. Multiple follicle cysts 3. Thick capsule	1. Multiple cortical cysts up to 1.5 cm. in diameter 2. Clear, serous fluid	1. Yellow-orange lined cyst 2. May be filled with clear, serous fluid 3. Hemorrhage frequent
Micro	1. Many cystic spaces 2. Fibrous, thick capsule	Cysts lined with follicular epithelium	1. Lined by large theca cells 2. Hemorrhage frequent
Special features	1. Bilateral wedge resection usually "cures" 2. May have low 17-beta-estradiol and increased 17-KS	1. *Most* common cyst of ovary; Laparotomy if symptomatic 2. 57% of all ovarian specimens in one series	1. Often present with hydatidiform mole or chorioepithelioma 2. 10% of all ovarian specimens in one series

OVARIAN TUMORS—GENERAL

1. Most ovarian tumors are *benign:*
   Total ovarian tumors 1740 cases
   Malignant ovarian tumors 265 (15%)
   Benign ovarian tumors 1475 (85%)
2. Most cystic tumors of ovary are *benign*
3. Cystic tumors of ovary are more common than solid ones
4. Higher percentage of solid ovarian tumors are malignant than cystic ovarian tumors

Benign vs. Malignant Serous Cystic Tumors

	Benign Serous Cystadenoma	*Malignant Serous Cystadenocarcinoma*
Origin	—————— Coelomic germinal (Müllerian) epithelium ——————	
General considerations	Comprise 25% of all ovarian tumors; benign:malignant ratio 2:1	
	20% bilateral Comprise 20% of all *benign* ovarian tumors	35% bilateral Comprise 65% of all *malignant* ovarian tumors
	May occur at any age, but usually between 20 and 50 yrs.	
Gross	—————— Usually large cysts, up to 30–40 cm., in diameter —————— —————— Smaller masses usually have a single cystic cavity —————— —————— Enlargement produces multilocularity and asymmetry ——————	
	Most have clear serous fluid Serosa smooth NO papillary projections	Small nodularities through serosa *Papillary projections*
Micro	Serous cells Single layer of cuboidal cells, *central* nucleus Some cells ciliated Some cells-dome-shaped, serous-secreting Psammoma bodies very rare in benign	Serous cells Piling up of epithelium Invasion of stroma/capsule of cyst Same type of cell as in benign form BUT anaplastic features Papillary formation Psammoma bodies COMMON

Mucinous Cystic Tumors

	(Pseudo) Mucinous Cystadenoma	(Pseudo) Mucinous Cystadenocarcinoma
Origin	Coelomic germinal (Müllerian) epithelium or gastrointestinal tract rest	
General considerations	——————— Benign/malignant ratio 7:1 to 9:1 ——————— ——————— Comprise 20% of all ovarian neoplasms ———————	
	25% of all benign ovarian tumors 5% bilateral	15% of all malignant ovarian tumors 20% bilateral
	Secretory product chemically similar to bowel and endocervical gland mucin, glairy mucus	
	Occurs mainly in adult life, *rarely* before puberty or after menopause	
Gross	Resemble serous cyst types, but tend to be much larger than serous	
	——————— More apt (than serous) to be unilateral ———————	
	Papillary formations much less common than in serous	
	Multiloculation more prominent than in serous	
Micro	Lining epithelium nonciliated, tall, columnar, mucus-secreting cells Nuclei—basal Mucoid secretion in luminal portion of cell	Piling up of epithelium Papillary formations Anaplasia, epithelial cells Invasion of capsule Formation of solid masses of tumor
Special features		Metastasis/rupture of cyst results in PSEUDOMYXOMA PERITONEI, which may also occur in mucocele of appendix Psammoma bodies and cilia not seen

Teratomas

	Cystic (Dermoid)	Solid (Complex)
Etiology	Parthenogenic ovarian rest	Embryonic rest
General	1. Usually less than 10 cm. diameter 2. Occurs in reproductive age group 3. Comprises 20% of all benign tumors 4. Lined by skin (dermoid) and adnexa	1. Often larger than dermoid 2. Occurs more often in prepubertal years 3. Comprises 1% of all malignant ovarian tumors 4. Similar to teratoma of testes
Gross	1. Smooth, glistening serosa 2. Filled with pultaceous material 3. Usually nipple area with hair follicles 4. Hair, teeth, bone	1. Smooth, glistening serosa with thick walls 2. Solid with foci of hardness 3. May have papillary excrescences 4. Cut surface = yellow/brown in tissue with tiny loculi and cystic spaces
Micro	1. Skin and adnexa 2. Cartilage, GI tract, bone, brain, etc.	1. Complete heterogeneity of adult structures 2. Tumor may have any pattern 3. Struma ovarii or chorioepithelium or carcinomatous or sarcomatous patterns may predominate
Special Features	1. Less than 1% of cystic teratomas are malignant 2. 97% of all ovarian teratomas are cystic 3. Rarely in walls of mucinous cystadenomas	1. 1% to 2% of all ovarian teratomas are solid 2. Most common in children; comprise about 15% of all ovarian tumors in children
	4. ————— Teratomas comprise 20% of all ovarian neoplasms —————	
	5. ————— 80% of teratomas are unilateral —————	

Solid Ovarian Tumors (Non-hormone-Producing)

Tumor	Benign to Malignant Ratio	Percentage of All Benign (Ovary) Tumors	Percentage of All Malignant (Ovary) Tumors	Bilateral	Features
Undifferentiated carcinoma	0:100	0%	10%	Often	Undifferentiated Grade IV tumor, prognosis hopeless
Fibroma	99.9:0.1	34%	0.28%	10%	Meigs' syndrome, 10%–20% right hydrothorax, ascites, ovarian fibroma
Brenner tumor	100:0	1.4%	0%	5%	1. Walthard cell rests 2. Associated with mucinous cystadenocarcinoma in 20% of cases
Dysgerminoma	0:100	0%	< 1%	15%	1. Micro same as seminoma in males 2. 20–30 age group most often 3. 5-year survival rate 30%
Krukenberg	0:100	0%	<1%	> 80%	1. Metastatic with primary in GIT 2. Signet-ring cells 3. Krukenberg ovary to GIT

Hormone-Producing Ovarian Tumors

	FEMINIZING		MASCULINIZING
	Granulosa-Cell Tumor	*Thecoma*	*Arrhenoblastoma*
Incidence	Uncommon (1.7% of all ovarian tumors) Benign/Malignant 66:33 Percent of all benign ovarian tumors 15% Percent of all malignant ovarian tumors 5% Percent bilateral 5%	Uncommon (2.2% of all ovarian tumors) Benign/malignant ratio = 100:0 Usually in older age group than granulosa-cell tumor, often mixed with granulosa-cell tumor	Less than 0.1% of all ovarian tumors Most benign, about 25% malignant or recur Occurs at any age from puberty to menopause
Micro	Geometric patterns = acinar and folliculoid Cylindroid Call-Exner bodies (resemble ovum-abortive follicle with acidophilic secretion)	Looks like fibroma with routine staining	Looks like male testis with interstitial cell hyperplasia, much variation in micro pattern
Gross	Usually 5–10 cm. in diameter; usually yellow in color		
Signs and symptoms	Same as thecoma	Depends on WHEN they occur Precocious puberty in children (boys start noticing baby sister) Menstrual life, often asymptomatic Postmenopausal, "mother blooms again"	Masculinization, deep voice, hirsutism, male distribution of hair, enlarged clitoris
Special features	Many feminizing ovarian tumors have some thecomatous (fibromatous) areas and some granulosa cell (geometric) areas; these tumors called granulosa-theca cell tumors	Fat stain (sudanophilic) differentiates from fibroma	Adrenal cortical tumors are much more common cause of hirsutism and masculinization than arrhenoblastoma

FALLOPIAN TUBES
SALPINGITIS

	Suppurative	*Tuberculous*
Etiology	Pyogenic organisms: *Neisseria gonorrhoeae* by far most common cause (90%); the rest due to streptococci, staphylococci, coliforms, *Clostridium welchii*	Tubes seeded hematogenously by TB bacilli (a secondary complication), 1%–2% of salpingitis
Signs and symptoms	Acute PID: lower abdominal pain, fever, dysmenorrhea, GI symptoms Chronic PID: pelvic pain, dysmenorrhea, adhesions may produce intestinal obstruction, sterility and tubal pregnancy often associated with chronic PID	May cause pain, dysmenorrhea, menstrual abnormalities
Gross	Acute PID: hyperemia and fibrin, lumen filled with pus, fimbriae sealed and distended tubes, "retort tubes" Chronic PID: a. Hydrosalpinx b. Salpingitis isthmica nodosa c. Obliterated tubes	Indistinguishable from chronic gonorrheal or pyogenic salpingitis
Micro	Acute PID: a. Intracellular gram-negative diplococci of GC (presumptive evidence) b. Polys c. Edema d. Granulation tissue Chronic PID: cysts, mononuclear cells, scarring, obstruction	Giant cells (Langhans' type). Fusion of mucosal folds with buried epithelial crypts (glandlike spaces)
Special Features	1. GC infection route via cervical canal, through endometrium, to tubes 2. Streptococcus infection route from a cervical or vaginal area via lymphatics and blood vessels to tubes	TBC salpingitis almost never occurs without history of pulmonary or gastrointestinal TBC

TUBAL PREGNANCY

Etiology

Obstruction of tube

Incidence

1/150 pregnancies; 95% of all ectopic (extrauterine) pregnancies

Signs and symptoms

1. Pain, usually in lower abdomen
2. "Bathroom" sign: fainted in bathroom, usually within 10–12 weeks
3. Tenderness in lower abdomen
4. Positive pregnancy test (UCG or Gravindex)

Gross

1. Enlarged tube, rounded mass, usually 2–3 cm. in diameter
2. Ruptures with hemorrhage
3. Fetus often present

Micro

1. Immature products of conception, must find villi or fetus to make a positive diagnosis
2. Inflammatory cells, RBC's, THIN

Special features

1. Late feature: necrosis, spontaneous regression or resorption of fetus if no rupture
2. Fetal retention with mummification (lithopedion) if no rupture
3. 2.5% of choriocarcinomas arise from ectopic pregnancies
4. 1 in 5,333 ectopic pregnancies becomes choriocarcinoma

TUMORS/CYSTS

Key words

Parovarian cysts/hydatids of Morgagni, very common, monolayers of flat epithelium line these

Carcinoma rare, adenocarcinoma pattern (picket-fence cells usually arise near fimbriated end)

Endosalpingosis uncommon, tubular epithelium deep in wall; may confuse with cancer, compare with direct endometriosis

27 Breast

ANATOMY AND HISTOLOGY OF THE BREAST

Connective Tissue

1. Periductal and intralobular connective tissue
2. Interlobular connective tissue

Epithelial Cells

1. Skin: keratinized stratified squamous epithelium
2. Ducts: columnar epithelium
3. Lobules: cuboidal epithelium

EMBRYOLOGY OF THE BREAST (MODIFIED SWEAT GLAND)

Appearance of the breast at various stages of life (two milk lines)
1. Birth: neonatal stage (maternal hormones), hyperplasia of ducts
2. Childhood: branching ducts and small epithelial buds. Hyperplasia, epithelial elements, interlobular, fibrous and adipose tissue
3. Adolescence: hyperplasia, age 12–16 female, male involution
4. Maturity: male quiescent (no lobules, ducts only). Female marked development of lobules, budding of ducts, hyperplasia of connective tissue
5. Menstrual Life: cyclic; hyperplasia of epithelium (estrogen); hyperplasia and edema of fibrous tissue, enlargement of blood vessels (progesterone); lymphocytes in stroma premenstrually.
6. Gestation: marked budding, hyperplasia of lobules with secretory activity
7. Lactation: hyperplasia and maturation of glands with apocrine secretion (colostrum, then milk), reversal of usual gland/stroma ratio, stromal edema also present.

THE BREAST AND HORMONES

Estrogen: ductal epithelium proliferation and budding in presence of growth hormone
Progesterone: lobular structures, stromal proliferation and edema in presence of growth hormone
Prolactin: lactation under influence of growth hormones, estrogen and progesterone

LYMPHATIC DRAINAGE (ROUTES OF METASTASIS)

1. Axillary and supraclavicular lymph node chain (most common route)
2. Groszman's path, directly backward through pectoralis major and minor

3. Through perforating branches of internal mammary nodes to mediastinal and pleural lymphatics
4. Paramammary route of Gerota (accounts for direct liver and upper abdominal metastases)
5. Lymphatics of skin across front of chest (explains tumor in opposite breast)

Hypertrophy of the Breast

	Male	*Female*
	1. Pubertal	1. Precocious mammary development
	2. Persistent pubertal	2. Infantile
	3. Senescent (hormonally active tumors)	3. Preadolescent
		4. Adolescent
	4. Gynecomastia—persistent enlargement of male breast (clinical term)	5. Gravid
		6. Postmenopausal (hormonally active ovarian tumors)
Etiology	Endocrine imbalance; nutritional deficiency; hormones (cirrhosis), most common cause	Response depends on hormones and end-organ response of breast tissue (e.g., receptor sites)
Histology	Hyperplasia of ducts, epithelial cells and myoepithelial cells, hyperplasia of periductal connective tissue	Hyperplasia of ducts, lobules and stroma

MAMMARY DYSPLASIA (FIBROCYSTIC DISEASE)

Definition

A group of lesions with similarities in:
1. Development: epithelial and stromal hormonal response
2. Clinical expression: bilateral, irregular breast masses
3. Histology: proliferation of ducts and/or stroma

Etiology

Hormonal imbalance (?) or altered end-organ response

Frequency

MOST common lesion of the breast of the *female;* 25–50% of all females show some evidence of it

Age

Peak age = last decade of reproductive life

Gross

Irregular, firm masses, usually bilateral, frequently in upper outer quadrant

Micro

1. Imperfect lobular development
2. Metaplasia (apocrine) of ductal epithelium (eosinophilic duct cells)
3. Hyperplasia of ductal epithelium
4. Incomplete involution of the hyperplastic ducts
5. Hyperplasia of fibrous stroma

6. Chronic inflammation, with lymphocytes, plasma cells, and histiocytes
7. Cyst formation

Variations

Mazoplasia: fibrosis and desquamation of the epithelium

Adenosis: (usually predominates in 35–45 age group); proliferation of ductal epithelium and connective tissue with marked fibrosis-sclerosing adenosis. May see intraductal papillomatosis and glandular duplication

Cystic Disease: (usually predominates in 45–55 age group); multiple cysts (blue dome)

Fibrous Dysplasia, also Called Mastodynia: (usually predominates in 30–35 age group); predominantly fibrous tissue with some inflammatory cells

Notes

1. Fourfold increase in incidence of breast cancer with mammary dysplasia; should biopsy all suspicious masses
2. Occasionally one pattern may predominate; then the patterns shown under "Variations" are seen, however, thorough examination will often reveal several patterns with most of the changes shown under "Micro" above in the same patient.

Benign Breast Tumors

	Fibroadenoma	*Intraductal Papilloma*
Etiology and pathogenesis	Hormonal stimulation: excess response; receptors (estrogen)	Unknown, some consider it a variant of fibrocystic disease
Frequency	3rd most common lesion of breast; most common benign tumor of female breast	Uncommon
Age	20–30 most common	Peak shortly before menopause
Location	Mostly upper outer quadrant, usually unilateral	Intraductal
Gross	Unilateral, firm, delicately encapsulated mass; gray-pink color	Firm, granular nodule; usually multiple

Micro	1. Epithelial hyperplasia
	2. Hyperplasia of connective tissue
	   a. pericanalicular
	   b. intralobular
		Delicate villous pattern, thin fibrovascular core with epithelium: 2 types of epithelial cells
		No cribriform pattern
		No invasion of stalk or base

Variations	1. Adenoma: fibroadenoma with scant fibrous proliferation 2. Giant fibroadenoma: (cystosarcoma phylloides)	Multiple or diffuse papillomatosis is similar
Gross	Bulky (often very large) tumor with rapid growth	

(Continued on opposite page)

Benign Breast Tumors *(continued)*

	Fibroadenoma	*Intraductal Papilloma*
Micro	Proliferation of epithelium, pseudo-sarcomatous proliferation of connective tissue, about 25% become malignant (fibrosarcoma)	Fewer stalk structures than simple papilloma
Special features	May be a variant of fibrous dysplasia	1. MOST common cause of bloody discharge from nipple; 50% of cases present with bloody discharge 2. Sclerosing adenosis frequent in adjacent breast tissue

Inflammations of the Breast

	Acute Mastitis	*Plasma Cell Mastitis*	*Chronic Mastitis*	*Fat Necrosis (Traumatic)*
Generalities	First few days of lactation (primigravida), uncommon in U.S.A.	Rare lesion, may mistake for cancer	Granulomatous inflammation (TB-syphilis-mycotic infection), very rare in U.S.A.	Most common in middle age; may mistake for cancer
Age		Peak incidence about 40; multigravida	Peak around menopause	
Etiology	Mostly *S. aureus*	Possible chemical-duct stasis; "split milk" mastitis	*M. tuberculosis* and others	Injury and necrosis of fat; left more common than right
Signs and symptoms	Inflammation	Pain, tenderness, distortion—retraction of nipple with discharge	"Lump," may resemble cancer	Dimpling and retraction, may resemble cancer
Gross	Cardinal signs of acute inflammation	Gray, mottled, with ectatic inspissated ducts on cut surface	Mass with necrosis	Early: firm, with fixation, with calcification and granulomatous response
Micro	Abscess and suppuration (acute inflammatory reaction)	Giant cells, plasma cells and foam cells; dilated ducts	Granulomas. Giant cells	Giant cells and chronic inflammation
Special features		Considered by some to be a variant of fibrocystic disease		

CARCINOMAS

Generalities

1. *ALL* are adenocarcinomas; approximately 90% are ductal, and 10% are lobular
2. Can occur at any age but most common around the menopause
3. Locations (in order of frequency):
   a. Upper outer quadrant (45%)
   b. Nipple and areolar area (25%)
   c. Upper inner quadrant (14%)
   d. Lower outer quadrant (10%)
   e. Lower inner quadrant (5%)
   f. Quadrant undetermined (1%)
4. MOST frequent fatal carcinoma in females
5. More common in nulliparous and primiparous than in multiparous females; more common with early menarche, cancer family history, long menstrual life (over 30 years)
6. Less common in mothers who nurse babies; more common in high socioeconomic group
7. Left:right ratio = 110:100
8. 0.5–2.0% are bilateral
9. Overall 5-year survival rate, 50% with surgery only
10. Prognosis poorer under 40 years of age

Noninfiltrating Intraductal Carcinoma

	Comedocarcinoma	Papillary Carcinoma
Definition	Malignant, solid growth, within duct, with central necrosis	Carcinoma with papillary structures confined to mammary duct systems
Incidence	Rare	Rare
Age	Postmenopausal	Any age group, but mostly 35–40
Clinical	Greasy, yellow-white nipple discharge, slow-growing	Bloody discharge from nipple, no fixation
Gross	No fixation with bulky, wormlike masses, nodular cut sections, greasy discharge	Well defined, segmental distribution, sometimes multiple Cut section: mammary of duct filled with pink, friable, gray-white tissue
Micro	Cellular cords with central necrosis, cribriform pattern and frequent mitotic figures Almost no stroma	Atypical papillary growth; no stalk, single type cell; cribriform pattern; no central necrosis Must differentiate from atypical papillary hyperplasia
Node metastasis	No	No
Prognosis	Cure with mastectomy	Cure with mastectomy

Infiltrating Ductal Carcinoma I

Scirrhous Carcinoma	Medullary Carcinoma	Paget's Disease	Mucinous (Colloid) Adenocarcinoma
Definition			
Adenocarcinoma of ducts with marked desmoplasia	Ductal adenocarcinoma with slight desmoplasia	Intraepithelial and central ductal Ca, resembling eczema	Mucin-producing ductal adenocarcinoma
Incidence			
75% of breast carcinomas	5%–10% of breast Ca	Over 5% of breast Ca	5% of breast carcinomas
Age			
50	45–50	Postmenopausal	Different ages
Clinical			
Hard mass with fixation (peau d'orange)	Large, soft mass	Long duration; eczematoid skin; burning, itching	Slow-growing, no fixation
Gross			
Usually 2–3 cm. mass, stony hard, fixed, infiltrating, gray appearance, chalky streaks, cuts like "unripe pear"	66% larger than 5 cm. deep location; soft, usually not fixed; central necrosis with hemorrhage	Eczematoid skin and oozing nipple	Soft, gelatinous, bulky, occasionally hemorrhagic, mass
Micro			
Marked hyaline fibrosis of stroma, "Indian-file" epithelial cells, areas of calcification	Large, bulky cells in sheets and cords; little fibrous tissue Lymphoid cells frequent	Intraepithelial (malignant) Paget's cells; central duct carcinoma	Multilocular; hyperplastic glands filled with basophilic (mucin-positive) amorphous material; seas of mucus with islands of cells or signet ring cells
Involvement of node			
66% have positive nodes	Usually negative	33% have nodes involved	33% have positive nodes

(Continued on overleaf)

Infiltrating Ductal Carcinoma I *(continued)*

Scirrhous Carcinoma	Medullary Carcinoma	Paget's Disease	Mucinous (Colloid) Adenocarcinoma
Prognosis			
50% 5-year survival; usually poor depending on node involvement and size of tumor mass; biologic predeterminism	70%–80% 5-year survival	Favorable if confined to nipple; rarely also Paget's is found in vulvar and axillary areas	76% 5-year survival without signet ring Almost hopeless with signet ring cells

Infiltrating Ductal Carcinoma II

Infiltrating Comedocarcinoma	Papillary Carcinoma	Inflammatory Carcinoma	Carcinoma of the Male Breast
Definition			
Malignant intraductal growth with central necrosis and infiltration	Malignant infiltrative papillary tumor	Invasive ductal Ca with subcutaneous lymphatic metastasis and signs of infiltration	Duplicates female except no lobular Ca Highly metastatic cancer
Incidence			
Under 10% of breast Ca	Under 5% of breast Ca	About 1% of breast Ca	Genetic factor, Klinefelter syndrome 100 × less common than in females
Age			
Postmenopausal	35–40 years	Young, 50% during lactation	
Clinical			
Cloudy nipple discharge; slow-growing	Bloody discharge from nipple, slow-growing	Signs and symptoms of inflammation	Bloody discharge
Gross			
Usually 5 cm., soft, pasty, cloudy discharge; fixation late, slightly circumscribed	5-cm., bulky tumor; central hemorrhage and necrosis	Firm, red, hot, edematous breast; induration of skin; central mass	

(Continued on opposite page)

Infiltrating Ductal Carcinoma II *(continued)*

Infiltrating Comedocarcinoma	Papillary Carcinoma	Inflammatory Carcinoma	Carcinoma of the Male Breast
Micro			
Cellular cords with central necrosis, cribriform pattern with invasion	Papillary structures; invasion into stroma; single cell type; cribriform pattern	Nonspecific Ca with subcutaneous lymphatic invasion; no inflammatory cells	Adenocarcinoma
Involvement of Node			
Seldom positive	Involved late	75% have nodes involved	
Prognosis			
75%–84% 5-year survival	80% 5-year survival	Poor	33% inoperable 30% 5-year survival

Malignant Epithelial Breast Tumors
LOBULAR CARCINOMA
(Mammary carcinoma arising in the lobule and terminal ducts)

	In Situ	Infiltrating
Age	29–83 (any age group) Peak 4th decade (45)	29–83 (any age group) Peak 4th decade (48)
Incidence	About 10% of total breast carcinomas	5% to 50% in situ
Gross	No definite gross appearance	Bulging lobules, tan color
Micro	Terminal ducts and lobules stuffed with plump epithelial cells; loss of cohesiveness and polarity; few mitotic figures	As in situ, plus infiltration of stroma by strands of neoplastic cells, may show Indian-file pattern
Location	Multiple origin, 66% upper outer quadrant	
Bilaterality	20–25%	75–80%
Prognosis	Cure with simple mastectomy	Varies depending on lymph node involvement Under 50% 5-year survival

28 Muscles, Bones, and Joints

Atrophy and Dystrophy of Muscle

	Muscle Atrophy	vs.	Muscular Dystrophy
Etiology	1. Loss of nerve supply 2. Anoxia		Primary, hereditary disease of muscle, several patterns
Gross	Small muscles with contracture late in course		Atrophy and pseudohypertrophy (due to fat and large muscle fibers)
Micro	Uniform shrinkage of muscle fibers in bundles, fibrous replacement later, increased sarcolemmal nuclei with perinuclear lipochrome, few lymphocytes, NO fat, normal muscle next to atrophic muscle		1. Pseudohypertrophy: swollen muscle fibers with fatty infiltration and vacuolar change 2. *Disorganized* mixture of shrunken and hypertrophic muscles, increased sarcolemmal nuclei
Special features	Most common cause is strokes; but can occur with any form of denervation or inflammation (e.g., dermatomyositis). Some may show special features such as central core myopathy		1. Duchenne (X-linked), pelvic girdle type, MOST common; waddling gait 2. Elevated CPK with MB and LDH with LDH$_1$. Also get SGOT and aldolase elevated 3. Increased urinary creatine and blood CPK

MALIGNANT TUMORS OF STRIATED MUSCLE

RHABDOMYOSARCOMA

Incidence

1. MOST common primary malignant tumor of muscle
2. 3rd most common malignant soft-tissue tumor
3. Younger children and adults usually affected
4. Common locations: uterus, kidney in children; extremities in older patients

Gross

Bulky fish flesh, sometimes focally hemorrhagic

Micro

3 Types
Undifferentiated: malignant spindle cells, giant cells frequent; "strap," basket, "stellate" cells, often hard to find cross striations

Alveolar: nests, may have glandlike structure
Embryonal: myxomatous (?) stroma

Special Features

1. MUST look for cross striations with (PTAH) stain
2. Also thought to be Wilms' kidney tumor and botryoid sarcoma in vagina of infants
3. MOST common primary malignant tumor of heart

MYASTHENIA GRAVIS

1. Muscle weakness, disease of foot plates (lack of acetylcholine, excess acetylcholinesterase) Rx'd by neostigmine, autoimmune disease (?)
   a. anti-cross striation antibodies 60–70% of patients
   b. anti-acetylcholine binding site antibodies frequent
2. Commonly associated with thymoma (20%) or hyperplasia of thymus (60%)
3. Most have NORMAL appearing muscle; lymphocytes may be present
4. More common in females
5. MOST commonly involved: extra-ocular and cranial nerve muscles
6. Micro of thymus: germinal centers in thymus (never normal in adults); epithelial cell tumor

MYOSITIS OSSIFICANS

	Circumscripta	*Progressiva*
Etiology	1. Most commonly due to TRAUMA 2. Probably from torn periosteum	Unknown, congenital (?). Most common in children
Definition	LOCALIZED hemorrhage and trauma into muscle with ORGANIZATION	GENERALIZED replacement of ALL soft tissue by bone
Gross	Firm, hard lesion of muscle	
Micro	Four zones: 1. Zone of hemorrhage 2. Zone of fibrosis 3. Cartilaginous zone 4. Zone of ossification	Three zones: NO zone of hemorrhage 1. Zone of fibrosis 2. Cartilaginous zone 3. Zone of ossification
Special features	Main problem: OFTEN mistaken for mesenchymal sarcoma	Usually begins in head and neck area Death due to muscle being replaced by bone

Some Common Tumors of Cartilage (Chondromas—Dyschondroplasias)

	Exostosis	Enchondroma	Chondrosarcoma
Incidence	Uncommon	Uncommon	Uncommon
Patient	Under 21	10–50 years of age	Older age group; Male 3:1
Common locations	Lower metaphysis of femur	Bones of hand	Common in bones of pelvis and long bones
Gross	Bone capped with cartilage	Cartilaginous growth	Large, whitish, firm, may have hemorrhagic area
Micro	Cartilage	Exuberant cartilage; ossification and calcification may be seen	Malignant cartilage cells 2 nuclei in each lacuna; may have bone spicules
Special features	Congential when multiple Really an osteoma Malignancy uncommon, but may occur	Ollier's disease when multiple Usually congenital Malignancy rare Maffucci's syndrome = enchondroma + hemagiomas of skin	Most common cause for hemipelvectomy Compare with osteogenic sarcoma Removal of primary tumor often causes rapid growth of metastases Prognosis better than other malignant sarcomas

Some Common Tumors of Bone

Osteogenic Sarcoma	Giant Cell Tumors	Ewing's Sarcoma
Incidence		
10–30 years of age Peak at 20 years, second peak at 60 years due to Paget's disease	Uncommon Mostly over 20 years of age No sex preponderance	Uncommon 10–30 years of age Slightly more common in males
Common locations		
Metaphysis of long bone: 1. upper tibia, 2. lower fibula, 3. upper humerus, 4. lower radius	Most common in upper end of tibia and lower end of femur	Medullary canal of metaphysis and diaphysis of long bones (50%) Innominate bone (20%)
Gross		
Mass in metaphysis of long bones Hard, white with bone formations	Usually in metaphysis of long bone Soft, curettable	Small, gray cystic areas; "onion skin" layering of periosteum on gross

(Continued on opposite page)

Some Common Tumors of Bone *(continued)*

Osteogenic Sarcoma	Giant Cell Tumors	Ewing's Sarcoma

Micro

Malignant cells with osteoid formation	Malignancy determined by stromal cells NOT giant cells	Sheets of small round cells, pseudorosettes

Special features

1. Most common primary malignancy of bone 2. Codman's triangle = elevation of periosteum 3. Alkaline phosphatase elevated 4. Ray markings on x-ray 5. 6% of osteogenic sarcomas arise in Paget's disease 6. 18% of Paget's disease develop into osteogenic sarcoma	Nonmalignant giant cell lesions: 1. Brown tumor of hyperparathyroidism 2. Giant cell granuloma of jaw (epulis)	Micro identical to: medulloblastoma, neuroblastoma, retinoblastoma

Prognosis

Poor	½ favorable outcome ½ recur after curetting 15% eventually need amputation 15% agressive and metastasize early	Very poor

Arthritis I

	Rheumatoid Arthritis (RA) vs.	Osteoarthritis (Degenerative)
Usual patient	Females (usually young) more common than males	Older age, males = females Most common type of arthritis overall, especially after 50 years of age
Etiology	Unknown, autoimmune (?); rheumatoid factor agglutinates latex; emotional stress (?)	Trauma, wear and tear Degeneration of cartilage
Common location	Small joints, most commonly the proximal interphalangeal joints of hands Ulnar deviation frequent Hepatosplenomegaly, lymphadenopathy with RA called Still's disease in children, Felty's syndrome in adults	Larger joints, knees, spine, (especially cervical), and terminal phalanges
Gross	Rheumatoid nodules in skin of 20% of patients	Bony spurs Lipping of spine
Micro	Proliferative granulation tissue	Degenerative changes

(Continued on overleaf)

Arthritis I *(continued)*

	Rheumatoid Arthritis (RA)	vs.	Osteoarthritis (Degenerative)
Special features	1. Amyloidosis (10%) 2. Pannus, anyklosis 3. Inflammation due to lysosomal breakdown when ingesting immune complex		1. Eburnation 2. Joint mice (bits of cartilage) 3. No pannus formation, no ankylosis 4. Heberden's nodes (calcific spurs) at bases of terminal phalanges
Complete crippling	20% of cases		Rare

ARTHRITIS II

Juvenile Rheumatoid Arthritis (JRA)

1. Etiology unknown; autoimmune (?) same as adult rheumatoid arthritis
2. Special features of JRA:
   a. The most common musculoskeletal disorder causing crippling in children
   b. The most common cause for childhood onset of blindness (due to chronic iridocyclitis)
   c. The most common underlying condition in amyloidosis in children
   d. 33% present as monarticular disease at the outset, usually in larger joints (most frequently in the knee)

Ankylosing Spondylitis

1. Formerly considered a variant of RA (RA test negative)
2. Usually involves spine—(males 9:1)
   Always involves sacroiliac joint, sometimes involves hip, shoulder, etc.
3. Now known to be associated with HLA B-27 tissue type antigen in high incidence
4. Pathology: synovitis and synovial hyperplasia, lymphocytes and plasma cells. Late: fibrosis (pannus), ankylosis, ossification, syndesmophytes on x-ray

Psoriatic Arthritis

1. Arthritis (RA test negative) associated with psoriasis
   More common in women than men
2. Three patterns are seen:
   a. Sacroiliitis
   b. Peripheral joints of hand with psoriasis in nails of hand
   c. Arthritis of several peripheral joints, usually asymmetrical
3. Pathology: synovial proliferation, round cells, scarring, ankylosis
4. Differentiate from RA: asymmetric, negative RA test, no subcutaneous nodules, but with psoriasis in skin

ARTHRITIS III

Reiter's Syndrome

1. Definition: nongonorrheal
   a. Arthritis
   b. Conjunctivitis,
   c. Urethritis and sometimes a mucocutaneous lesion on glans penis
2. Most frequently seen in young men ages 20–40 years.

3. Etiology: unknown, suspect chlamydias
4. Pathology: villous hyperplasia, and round cells in synovium to pannus formation

Gastrointestinal Associated Arthridites

A. Ulcerative colitis (UC)
    1. 20% of UC patients develop an arthritis—usually in a single peripheral joint, knee, ankle, foot. The spine can be involved.
    2. Pannus and ankylosis occur but are uncommon
B. Regional enteritis
    1. Under 5% have arthritis
    2. Pattern similar to UC

Arthritis IV

	Suppurative vs.	*Tuberculous*
Usual patient	Male 10–30 years	TB patient with pulmonary TB
Etiology	Blood-borne MOST common route Direct trauma 2nd most common route Gonococcus Staphylococcus Streptococcus (*S. pneumoniae*)	*Mycobacterium tuberculosis*
Common locations	Large joints Knee, hip Usually monarticular	Spine = Pott's disease, most common
Gross	Hot, red, swollen, painful	Cold, swollen
Micro	Polys to healing with scar and ankylosis	Langhans' giant cells Caseous necrosis
Special features	Amyloidosis with long-standing infection Pannus infrequent	Amyloidosis may occur Pannus formation may occur More destructive than suppurative arthritis

Osteomyelitis

	Pyogenic	vs.	Tuberculous
Etiology	Most common by hematogenous route Organisms (order of frequency): staphylococcus, streptococcus, *S. pneumoniae* and others		*M. tuberculosis* most common; secondary to pulmonary TBC
Incidence and clinical	Uncommon now Boys 3:1 girls More common in children		Uncommon now More common in children than in adults
Symptoms	Four cardinal signs of inflammation		Usually NO heat
Pathology	Most common location to begin: narrow cavity of metaphyses of long bones (order of frequency): femur, tibia, humerus Get polys, then sequestrum (dead bone) and involucrum (newly forming bone)		Much more destructive than pyogenic osteomyelitis Most common locations (order of frequency): Spine (Pott's disease), long bones
Micro			Same as TBC elsewhere
Complications	1. Sinus tracts 2. Suppurative arthritis (knee most common) 3. With long-standing chronic osteomyelitis secondary amyloidosis is common 4. Brodie's abscess: chronic infection/sterile		1. Persistence: harder to control than pyogenic osteomyelitis 2. TBC arthritis if a joint is involved 3. Psoas (cold) abscess with Pott's disease

FRACTURE HEALING

Sequence of Events
1. Hemorrhage: RBC, WBC, and plasma proteins exuded into area
2. Coagulation: a fibrin meshwork forms, serves as scaffold for fibroblasts, then lyses
3. Acute and then chronic inflammatory cells invade and start clearing up debris
4. Granulation tissue grows in, fibrin mesh lyses as collagen is laid down
5. Cartilage is laid down
6. Osteoid is formed
7. Calcification: provisional procallus, formed around fracture
8. Final healing: remodeling, rearrangement of bone spicules and loss of procallus, cannot tell from new bone

Complications
1. Pseudoarthrosis: inadequate mobilization
2. Angulation
3. Shortening
4. Poor healing: nonunion, especially hip area

Common Dwarfs

	Pituitary	Achondroplastic	Cretin
Basic defect	Lack of growth hormone	Failure of normal endochondral bone formation and premature closing of epiphyses, Mendelian dominant	Congenital lack of thyroid hormone in utero and after birth. Hypoplasia of thyroid gland
Description	Angelic, childlike stature	Circus dwarf	Myxedema
Head	Small	Large	Large
Extremities	Long	Short	Short, curved arms
Trunk	Small	Large	Short
Special features	Hypogonadism	Hypergonadism Lumbar lordosis Intramembranous bone formation is normal	Hypogonadism, mental retardation; pot belly, umbilical hernia, thick lips, protruding tongue, dry skin, coarse hair
Micro	Normal, slow growth	Disarray of endochondral bone columns at epiphyses with thin zones of cartilage cells	Lack of growth

MISCELLANEOUS MUSCULOSKELETAL DISEASES: KEY WORDS

Baker's Cyst

Nonneoplastic herniation of knee joint into popliteal space

Chordoma

1. Tumor of notochord; very rare
2. Occurs at basisphenoidal and sacrococcygeal areas of cord
3. Micro: physaliferous cells

Fibrous Dysplasia (Monostotic and Polyostotic)

1. Fibrous overgrowth of bony trabeculae without internal lamellar structure, etiology unknown
2. Albright's syndrome
   Polyostotic fibrous dysplasia
   Melanotic skin pigmentation
   Precocious puberty in young females
3. Monostotic much more common than polyostotic form

Ganglion

1. Cystic swelling of tendon sheath
2. Most common over wrist

Gargoylism (Hurler's Disease)

1. Hepatosplenomegaly, mental retardation, blindness due to cataracts; gargoyle-like head
2. Basic defect—abnormal lysosomal storage of mucopolysaccharides in histiocytes in liver and glycolipids in brain
3. Autosomal recessive, alpha-L-iduronidase lacking

Hunter's Syndrome

Same as Hurler but NO cataracts; lack of iduronyl-2-0-sulfatase

Osteitis Deformans (Paget's Disease of Bone)

1. Most common in old age
2. More common in males 2:1
3. Bone process :replacement of normal bone by thick, soft, poorly mineralized bone in "mosaic pattern"; highest alkaline phosphatase of any disease
4. 10% to 20% of cases develop into osteogenic sarcoma

Osteogenesis Imperfecta (Fragilitas Ossium)

1. Brittle bones, blue sclera
2. Usually present at or soon after birth
3. Uncommon hereditary disease, usually autosomal dominant
4. Generalized defect in synthesis of connective tissue
5. Otosclerosis (deafness) commonly associated

Osteopetrosis (Albers-Schonberg Disease)

1. "Marble bone" disease
2. Key process : overgrowth and sclerosis of bone with little or no marrow cavity
3. Extramedullary hematopoiesis, blindness, deafness, and cranial nerve paralysis due to bony overgrowth
4. Autosomal recessive inheritance

Pigmented Villonodular Synovitis

1. Chronic inflammatory lesion with hemosiderin-laden macrophages (yellow) in synovia
2. Most common in knee joint of athlete
3. Have frondlike projections into joint, giant cells common
4. On finger, called giant cell tumor of tendon sheath origin, "fingeroma"
5. May be mistaken for malignancy; is not

Synoviosarcoma

1. Rare tumor
2. Occurs in middle to late adult life
3. Most common in lower extremities
4. Cleftlike space lined with cuboidal epithelium
5. May confuse with pigmented villonodular synovitis

29 Reticuloendothelial System

Chronic Lymphadenitis

	Nonspecific	Dermatopathic
Etiology, pathogenesis, and clinical	1. Associated with chronic inflammation and trauma 2. The MOST common finding in lymph nodes 3. Most common and most severe in inguinal nodes 4. Nontender nodes	1. Associated with chronic dermatoses and scratching 2. Eczema, psoriasis, exfoliative dermatitis, seborrheic dermatitis, etc.
Gross	Firm, white nodes, normal sized or slightly enlarged	Firm, moderately enlarged yellow-brown colored lymph nodes, black periphery occasionally seen
Micro	1. Enlarged germinal centers 2. Increased lymphocytes and histiocytes 3. Macrophages with phagocytosed debris 4. "sinus catarrh," free histiocytes and lymphocytes in sinuses 5. Fibrosis, scar	1. Nodular: follicular hyperplasia and reticulum cells (histiocytes); cells often in sheets 2. Accumulation of melanin and hemosiderin in macrophages (histiocytes) 3. Lipid droplets in macrophages 4. Little fibrosis usually
Special features	1. DO NOT biopsy inguinal nodes when looking for lymphomas 2. Note the "specific" lymphadenitides, such as TB and sarcoidosis, are covered in appropriate sections of *The Bare Facts of General Pathology* by Joseph A. Sisson. Ed.2. Philadelphia, J.B. Lippincott, 1974.	1. DO NOT mistake for lymphoma or melanoma

Anatomic Pathology of Chronic Leukemias

	Granulocytic	Lymphocytic	Monocytic
Age range	Usually in middle age	Older adult	Middle age
Cells	Abnormal, immature granulocytes	Small abnormal lymphocytes (B cells)	Abnormal monocytes with "football" nucleus
Spleen size	LARGEST of any disease, to 5000 g.	Large (2500 g.)	Moderately large, to 1000 g.
Cut surface	Firm, yellow, maplike, loss of follicular pattern	Firm, white-gray, loss of follicular pattern	Firm, moderate preservation of follicular pattern
Lymph node	1+	4+	1+
	All cause homogeneous soft, white FISH FLESH appearance in nodes		
Liver size	1+	4+ (biggest liver of all)	1+
Cut surface	Diffuse infiltrate	Focal white nodules	Infiltrate diffuse if present
Special features	Leukemias are one of 4 most common tumors involving the heart		
	Philadelphia chromosome commonly present, Auer rods	Christchurch chromosome uncommonly present	Commonly involves the gums
Prognosis	Poor (3 years), usually progresses to acute leukemia	Good, 6 years average survival	POOREST, under 3 years

Anatomic Pathology of Acute Leukemias

In general, they have such a rapid course with hemorrhagic and systemic symptoms that there is usually little or often NO significant spleen or liver enlargement.

	Granulocytic	Lymphocytic	Monocytic
Key clinical features	Most common in middle age	Most common in children	Most common in middle age
Prognosis	Poor	Poor	Poor
Key cell	Myeloblast, Auer rods common but not pathognomonic	Lymphoblast, "T" cell No Auer rods	Monoblast in pure monocytic Myeloblast and monoblast in mixed Auer rods uncommonly present

HAIRY CELL LEUKEMIA

1. Cell of origin considered to be either lymphocyte or monocyte (histiocyte)
2. Cells have hairlike projections on peripheral smear.
3. Cells contain tartrate-resistant acid phosphatase (Fraction 5)
4. Prognosis good with splenectomy
5. Dry bone marrow tap frequent

Malignant Lymphomas—I

	Lymphocytic Lymphoma		Histiocytic Lymphoma (Reticulum Cell Sarcoma)
	(Lymphoblastoma) Poorly Differentiated	*(Lymphosarcoma) Well Differentiated*	
Clinical	Most common in young adults	Biphasic, most common in childhood and old age; rare in young adults	Older age adults
Relative occurence	30% to 40% of all lymphomas		10% of all lymphomas
Gross	Lymph nodes, fish flesh, enlarged, white; NO fusion of nodes or attachment to other structures	Enlarged, white, fish flesh; pink nodes with rare fusion or matting	Large, matted, white, fish flesh lymph node with extension to adjacent structures
Micro	Obliteration of normal node outline with immature lymphoblasts, often with indented, lobulated nuclei	Obliteration of normal node architecture with normal mature looking lymphocytes "lymphosarcoma cell"	1. Large, bizarre histiocytes with large vesicular nuclei 2. Reticulum fibers around each cell or small group of cells
Special features	May be a variant of immunoblastoma	The second most common primary tumor of stomach and small intestine	Cells may be found to be lymphoblasts instead of histiocytes
Prognosis	Good (to 10-yr. survival)	Good in old people (to 15 yrs.) Poor in children	Poor (1–2 yrs.)

Malignant Lymphomas—II

Jackson and Parker =	*Hodgkin's Paragranuloma*	*Hodgkin's Granuloma*	*Hodgkin's Sarcoma*
Lukes et al. =	*Lymphocyte Predominant*	*Nodular Sclerosing (NS) Mixed Cellularity (MC)*	*Lymphocyte Depletion*
Prognosis	Good 90% 5-yr. survival	Fair 30% 5-yr. survival	Poor 1 to 2-yr. survival
Frequency	20%	40% NS; 25% MC	15%
Pathology Gross	Enlarged nodes	Enlarged, mottled nodes, suet pudding spleen	Large, mottled lymph nodes
Micro	Diffuse lymphocytic infiltration, RARE Reed-Sternberg cells, NO necrosis, eosinophils or fibrosis	Classic granulomas, Reed-Sternberg cells, lymphocytes, lacunar cells, fibrosis, eosinophils	Large reticulum cells with many Reed-Sternberg cells, rare to NO lymphocytes
Special features	1. Basic defect in Hodgkin's disease now considered to be T cell deficiency: patients have no response to T cell antigen (e.g., anergic) 2. Melbourne chromosome (MI) positive in some cases of Hodgkin's disease of any type 3. Spleen shows suet pudding pattern in Hodgkin's disease		

Lymphomas and Hodgkin's Disease Staging

Stage	Definition	Prognosis (5-year survival) (for Hodgkin's disease)
I	Disease localized to one area	90%
II	Disease in 2 areas on 1 side of diaphragm	85%
III	Disease on both sides of diaphragm	65%
IV	Visceral level, spleen, liver, or bone marrow involved	35%
A = No systemic symptoms B = Systemic symptoms		

Lymphocytic Lymphoma vs. Hodgkin's Disease

	Lymphocytic Lymphoma	*Hodgkin's Disease*
Age at onset	Occurs at extremes of life	Peak ages 18–38 yrs., rare at puberty
Usual method of presentation	Asymptomatic with symmetrically involved cervical lymph node	Asymptomatic (or with pruritus) with asymmetric enlarged cervical nodes
Pruritus	Rare	May precede, frequently accompanies
Fever	Rare early in disease	Pel-Ebstein, frequent
Lesion	Common in upper respiratory passages or GIT	Rare in upper respiratory passages or GIT

(Continued on opposite page)

Lymphocytic Lymphoma vs. Hodgkin's Disease *(continued)*

	Lymphocytic Lymphoma	Hodgkin's Disease
Lymph node		
Involvement	Usually symmetrical	Usually asymmetrical
Cervical	Usually bilateral	Usually unilateral
Sternal	Rarely involved	Commonly involved
Epitrochlear	May be involved	Almost never involved
Response to radiation	Immediate	Delayed

Malignant Lymphomas—III

	Giant Follicle (Nodular) Lymphoma vs.	Undifferentiated Stem Cell Lymphoma
Clinical	1. Usually begins in one node 2. Usually occurs from middle to older age 3. Some believe it is a variant of any lymphoma, others believe it is a separate entity	1. Burkitt's lymphoma is a specific variant 2. Most common involvement—jaw and internal organs, particularly ovary 3. Usually in children 4. Most common in Africa, but worldwide in distribution 5. Epstein-Barr virus probably etiologic
Gross	Spleen enlarged, accentuates malphigian pattern; "too many, too large"	Unilaterally enlarged jaw and abdominal mass
Micro	Giant follicle distributed evenly throughout cortex and medulla, cracking off; artefact; fading of follicles at edge; no evidence of inflammation	Uniform lymphocytes with "starry sky" histologic pattern due to lacunar cells (modified histiocytes)
EM	Dendritic cells with desmosomes between tumor cells	Nuclear projections with polar aggregates of mitochondria
Prognosis	Best of all lymphomas, to 20 years if it does not progress to another form of lymphoma	Chemotherapy produces dramatic results and some durable remissions ("cures")

CURRENT CONCEPTS OF IMMUNE SYSTEM REACTIONS

Introduction:

Along with expansion of our knowledge of the "B" and "T" effector cells of the immune system has emerged a group of diseases which range from hyperplasia of the normal immune system to frank malignancy of the system, currently called immunoblastic sarcoma. This concept has also cast some doubt over the current classification of some of the malignant lymphomas. The essentials of the current but rapidly changing concept of this spectrum of diseases are shown below.

	Benign Immunoblastic Response	Angioimmunoblastic Lymphadenopathy Immunoblastic Lymphadenopathy	Immunoblastic Sarcoma
Etiology	1. Immunization: foreign antigens (e.g., vaccinia and other viruses) 2. Drugs: penicillin, anticonvulsants 3. Autoimmunity: lupus, rheumatoid arthritis	? "Abnormal" response to foreign or autoantigens	1. Prolonged exposure to antigenic stimuli 2. Abnormal immune status (e.g., lupus)
Pathogenesis	"Normal" response to foreign or autoantigens	Abnormal reaction of B cells	Malignant response or degeneration of immune cells
Clinical findings	Asymptomatic or fever, malaise; generalized or localized lymphadenopathy	Fever, sweats, weight loss, generalized lymphadenopathy and polyclonal Age range usually 40–60 years M:F ratio nearly equal	
Gross	Large, firm, homogeneous, not matted nodes	Large, firm, gray, not matted nodo	Large, firm, gray, matted node
Micro	1. Nodular (follicular) B-cell and/or diffuse (interstitial) T-cell hyperplasia 2. Mixed cell proliferation includes plasma cells, eosinophils and immunoblasts 3. Vascular proliferation or arborization occasionally seen	Key TRIAD ("sine qua non") 1. Proliferation or arborization of small vessels 2. Prominent immunoblasts (transformed lymphocytes) proliferation with plasmacytoid lymphocytes and plasma cells 3. Deposition of amorphous interstitial material	1. Monomorphous: proliferation of abnormal hyperplastic immunoblasts 2. Occasionally plasma cell and plasmacytoid cells are seen
Special comments	Sometimes difficult to differentiate from malignant lymphoma	Median survivial = 15 months	Survivial usually under months
Note	There are many variants with various names being proposed. This whole area is currently in a great state of flux.		

LYMPHOMAS AND DYSPROTEINEMIA

Generalities:

It has been suggested that many malignant lymphomas arise from B cells of the immune series (immunoblasts). Evidence for this is based on two things so far: Morphological: e.g. plasma cells or plasmacytoid lymphocytes in lesion with lateralized nucleus, coarse, clumped chromatin, perinuclear halo and cytoplasmic basophilia. Serum protein studies associated with lymphomas

The following is a summary of the current status of this subject:

Cytologic Patterns of "Lymphomas" Associated With Dysproteinemia

	Classic Malignant Lymphomas	Plasma Cell Diseases	Lesions with Appearance Similar to Lymphomas but with Excess Plasmacytoid Cells
Diseases	Classic lymphomas: stem cell. Lymphocytic Hodgkin's, etc.	Benign monoclonal gammopathy to myeloma	Lymph node hyperplasia, immunoblastic lymphoma, Immunoblastic sarcoma
Frequency of abnormal protein	Sometimes but not always present	Usually an "M" protein in serum and often Bence-Jones protein in urine	Frequently show polyclonal gammopathy
Immunoglob-ulin type	Usually IgM	Usually IgG	Usually IgG
Notes	Hodgkin's with nodular pattern is least likely to produce immunoglobulins	May have IgM, IgG, IgA, IgD, IgE	Usually IgG or IgM, sometimes mixed

DISEASES OF THE SPLEEN—KEY WORDS

Accessory Spleen

1. 10% of population
2. Most common at spleen hilus

Amyloidosis (Secondary)

1. Sago spleen (white pulp)
2. Lardaceous spleen (red pulp)

Chronic Passive Congestion

1. Most common lesion of spleen, 99% of patients
2. More severe with portal hypertension due to cirrhosis

Fleckmilz of Feitis (Speckled Spleen)

Found in areas of necrosis in spleen; associated with septicemia or uremia

Gamna-Gandy Bodies (Blue-Fabric Lesion)

1. Gross: brown specks in enlarged uniform spleen
2. Micro: prussian-blue positive, hemosiderin
3. Most commonly hemosiderin seen in spleen in severe CPC with hemorrhage or in long-standing hemolytic disease

Infarcts

1. Common
2. Usually due to emboli from left side of heart
3. End-organ circulation, white infarct
4. Frequent with polycythemia and sickle cell anemia

Infectious Mononucleosis (IM)

1. Spleen enlarged
2. Ruptured spleen most common cause of death in mono
3. IM most common predisposing cause of ruptured spleen

Miliary Nodules

1. Calcified, millet-seed nodules
2. In about 50% of all autopsies on persons over 50 yrs.
3. Old TBC most common etiology

Myeloid Metaplasia (Extramedullary Hematopoiesis)

1. All bone marrow elements found in spleen
2. Spleen most common site, liver is second
3. Usually due to bone marrow replacement
4. Myelophthisic anemia most commonly with fibrous tissue, called myelofibrosis
5. Teardrop RBC's in peripheral smear are most characteristic

Effects of Splenectomy

1. Transitory
   Anemia or polycythemia
   Severe leukocytosis
   Normal platelet count
   Abnormal RBC morphology: target cells, nucleated RBC's, Howell-Jolly bodies
2. Long-term
   RBC's: abnormal morphology, Howell-Jolly bodies are most characteristic
   WBC's: slight to moderate leukocytosis
   Platelets: usually normal, thrombocytopenia in 33% with increased incidence of thromboembolism

Hypersplenism (Enlarged Spleen)

1. Also called congestive splenomegaly
2. Leukopenia
3. Anemia
4. Thrombocytopenia

Tumor Metastases

Uncommon: (theories- a. infertile soil; b. penicilliary artery, trapping)

30 CNS–Vascular Diseases and Trauma

GENERALITIES OF ANATOMY AND PATHOLOGY

Neurons of the Central Nervous System

1. Neurons of the CNS are postmitotic (G_O) cells and never undergo mitosis
2. Nuclei: large and vesicular
3. Cytoplasm contains Nissl substance (rough endoplasmic reticulum) and neurofibrils, which are best stained with silver
4. Reaction of peripheral neurons to injury: axonal (Wallerian) degeneration
   Cut nerve fiber and get:
   a. Degeneration of myelin sheath and neurofibrils of entire distal segment and proximal segment to next node of Ranvier; complete in about 12 days
   b. Nissl degeneration, loss of Nissl substance and rounding of cell body by 12–24 hours
   c. Peripheral displacement of nucleus by 12–24 hours
   d. Regeneration, 1st Schwann cells synthesize myelin sheath; then neurofibrils grow out at slow rate
   e. Can get amputation neuroma at end of myelin if nerve ends are not properly aligned; phantom (?) limb syndrome

"Scars" of the CNS

"Scars" in the CNS are caused by GLIAL proliferation; more properly called "gliosis"; true fibroblasts found in brain only in brain abscesses and metastatic tumors

Virchow-Robin Space

1. Artefact of routine histologic processing
2. Represents astrocytic foot processes
3. Enlarged in cerebral edema and helpful in its diagnosis

CEREBRAL EDEMA

Clinical

Headache, papilledema, vomiting, convulsions, abducens palsy
Plain X-ray may show atrophy of sella turcica and inner table of skull; shifted pineal body, visible if calcified

Pathology

Gross:
1. Flattening of gyri, narrowing of sulci
2. Heavy weight (over 1400 g.)
3. Herniation
   Cingulate gyrus and falx cerebri in unilateral cerebral lesion
   Uncal (under tentorium cerebelli)
   Cerebellar tonsillar (into foramen magnum)
4. Duret hemorrhages in pons and medulla

Micro:
1. Enlarged Virchow-Robin spaces
2. Enlarged perinuclear halos of oligodendroglia

CNS DISEASE AS A CAUSE OF SUDDEN DEATH

1. In general, CNS diseases do NOT cause SUDDEN death (death in less than 1 hr. after onset)
2. Only CNS diseases that can cause sudden death are massive hemorrhage, trauma, or infarcts involving pons and medulla (respiratory and cardiac centers)
3. Most patients with even massive strokes live for 12 to 24 hours
4. MOST common causes of sudden death in USA are:
   Myocardial infarction (heart attack) with arrhythmia
   Trauma due to automobile accident or others
5. Airway obstruction is another, but probably not very common, cause of sudden death

CNS CELLS

Generalities
1. Cannot see cytoplasm of glial cells with usual H and E stains unless a pathologic process is present
2. Must be able to identify cells by their nuclei

	Astrocyte	*Oligodendroglia*
Nuclei	Large, round, vesicular	Small, round, compact with perinuclear halo
Function	1. Foot processes abut on blood vessels 2. Support CNS	1. Synthesize myelin 2. Homologue of Schwann cell in PNS
Normal arrangement	Random	Satellites to neurons, in streaming rows; most numerous glial cells
Reaction in pathologic conditions	1. *Gemistocytic:* plump, red cytoplasm with H and E in infarcts or around abscesses 2. *Proliferate:* gliosis "scar" in area of infarcts or abscess 3. *Malignant:* astrocytomas	1. *Satellitosis:* around damaged neurons 2. *Neuronophagia* (pseudoneuronophagia): indenting of damaged neuronal cytoplasm 3. *Malignant:* oligodendrogliomas
Histogenesis	Neuroectoderm	Neuroectoderm

	Microglia	Ependymal Cells	Endothelial Cells
Nuclei	Small, tricornuate, compact	Small, round, compact	Small, elongated, compact
Function	1. Phagocytic (RE system) endothelial cells 2. Support CNS	1. Line ventricles 2. Secrete (?) CSF	1. Line lumina of blood vessels 2. Tight junctions of these cells considered to be "blood-brain barrier"
Normal arrange-ment	Random	Glandlike; around ventricles	Around blood vessels

Reaction in pathologic conditions	1. *True digestion* of injured neurons
	2. Become *gitter cells;* plump with ingested debris in area of necrosis
	3. Gitter cells also from macrophages in blood
		1. *Proliferate:* in chronic inflammation, ependymitis granularis, syphilis
		2. *Flattened:* hydrocephalus
		3. *Malignant:* ependymoma may form blepharoplasts
			1. *Proliferate*
			  a. In area of gliosis
			  b. In tumor areas

Histogenesis	Mesoderm	Neuroectoderm	Mesoderm

PERTINENT CONGENITAL DEFECTS—I: KEY WORDS

Porencephaly

Abnormal cone-shaped opening of ventricles to meninges of cerebral surface

Rachischisis (Spina Bifida)

Failure of closure of posterior portion of spinal canal; asymptomatic without cord or meningeal herniation

Spina Bifida Occulta

Incomplete closure of posterior spinal canal usually asymptomatic; no protrusion of cord or meninges; local overlying hirsutism and hyperpigmentation common

Meningocele

Spina bifida with meninges herniated into a sac; most common in sacral area

Meningomyelocele

Spina bifida with meninges and spinal cord herniated into a sac; most common in sacral area

Dysrhaphia

Defective and/or lack of fusion of borders of neural groove; anencephaly is most severe form; spina bifida occulta is least severe

Platybasia

Flattened angle of dorsum sellae and clivus; often associated with narrowing of foramen magnum and fusion of odontoid processes of atlas to occipital bone; most commonly congenital, but may be caused by rickets or Paget's disease

	Arnold-Chiari Malformation	*Klippel—Feil Malformation*
Definition	1. *Arnold:* elongation of cerebellar tonsils into foramen magnum, with or without hydrocephalus; with or without associated spina bifida, meningocele, meningomyelocele 2. *Chiari:* elongation of medulla oblongata with deformity of lumbosacral cord without internal hydrocephalus 3. *Arnold-Chiari:* both of above with internal hydrocephalus due to obstruction of foramina of Luschka and Magendie—compression and elongation of 4th ventricle 4. Platybasia commonly associated	Abnormal fusion in utero of cervical vertebrae with shortened neck Asymptomatic by itself Associated conditions: a. Syringomyelia (common) b. Spina bifida (common) c. Mental defects: congenital deafness and squint are less commonly associated
Etiology	1. Unknown 2. Shortened spinal cord (?)	
Special features	10%–20% of meningomyeloceles have Arnold-Chiari malformations	Clinically "mirror image movements" in contralateral upper extremities are common
Symptoms	Usual onset in early childhood; rarely asymptomatic until adult life	
Prognosis	Better with late onset; poorer with childhood onset	

Hydrocephalus

	Internal (Noncommunicating) Obstructive	*External (Communicating) Nonobstructive*
Etiology and pathogenesis	*Infants:* 1. Most common stenosis of aqueduct of Sylvius 2. Arnold-Chiari - 2nd 3. Meningitis, pyogenic, TB, toxoplasmosis 4. Congenital stenosis of Luschka and Magendie, very rare *Adults:* 1. Tumors, focal common (colloid cyst of 3rd ventricle, rare) 2. Meningitis, especially TBC	1. Excess secretion of CSF by choroid plexuses 2. Lack of resorption of CSF by arachnoid villi and meninges 3. Trauma and hygroma or hematoma cause excess fluid in subdural space, especially focally
Clinical	Infants: large head, small face, no closure of sutures or fontanelles Adults: headache, cranial nerve palsies, (fainting with change in position of head = colloid cyst of 3rd ventricle) and signs of increased intracranial pressure	
Dye	*Does not* pass from lateral ventricle to spinal CSF	*Does* pass from lateral ventricle to spinal CSF
Special features	Hydrocephalus ex vacuo; accumulation of excess fluid without increased pressure in ventricles with atrophy of brain; most common in old people with senile brain atrophy; can occur with any degenerative CNS disease	

Arterial Causes of Infarctions of the Brain

	Thrombosis	Embolism	Intracerebral Hemorrhage
Etiology and pathogenesis	Occlusion by thrombus superimposed on arteriosclerotic artery	Occlusion by thromboembolism from left heart or elsewhere; most common cause is mural thrombus	1. Rupture of intracerebral artery almost always secondary to hypertension 2. Common with overdose of dicumarol
Incidence	50% of all strokes 90% of all occlusive strokes	Less than 10% of all strokes Less than 10% of occlusive strokes	40% of all strokes
Clinical	1. Generally abrupt onset of stroke, often during sleep or within 1 hr. of arising 2. Transient warning Sx common 3. Headache, rare 4. CSF usually normal	1. Most rapid onset of full-blown syndrome in seconds or minutes, onset anytime 2. No transitory warning Sx 3. Headache uncommon 4. CSF usually normal	1. *Gradual:* (1–6 hrs.) onset of syndrome 2. No warning symptoms 3. Headaches frequent and severe 4. CSF: usually RBC's and xanthochromia
Gross	Swollen, soft brain, secondary hemorrhage may occur *Locations:* a. Middle cerebral (65%) b. Carotid artery (17%) c. Vertebral and basilar (7%) d. Posterior cerebral (7%) e. Anterior cerebral artery (4%)	Hemorrhage may occur *Locations:* most common in smaller branches of a. Middle cerebral artery b. Anterior cerebral artery c. Posterior cerebral artery	Massive hemorrhage *Locations:* a. Cerebral hemispheres and basal ganglia (80%) b. Pons and midbrain (10%) c. Cerebellar (10%)
Micro	12–24 hrs.: neuronal and oligodendroglial degeneration, cytoplasmic staining, chromatolysis, pyknosis, Nissl lysis and edema 24–48 hrs.: edema with polys as predominant cells 72–96 hrs.: gitter cells gradually take over Late: gitter cells and gliosis		Massive hemorrhage and cerebral edema; rarely long survival; if do survive get same micro as thrombosis with hemosiderin-laden gitter cells
Special features	1. Symptoms depend on artery affected (see syndromes of cerebral arteries) 2. Lowest mortality rate of all strokes	1. Stokes-Adams syndrome (asystole over 10 secs. causes unconsciousness) 2. Carotid-vertebral angiography spasm (?), xenoembolic syndrome; usually transient, may be permanent 3. Second highest mortality rate of all strokes	1. Sudden death ONLY if massive medullary and pontine hemorrhage 2. Highest mortality rate of all strokes 3. Coin hemorrhages, leukemia

SOME SYNDROMES OF THE CEREBRAL ARTERIES

Anterior Cerebral Artery Syndrome

Paralysis and cortical hypesthesia of opposite lower extremities; mental changes (frontal lobe), incontinence (bowel-bladder); if Heubner's artery (to anterior perforated space) on dominant side is involved get aphasia because it supplies subcortical white matter of Broca's speech area

Basilar Artery Syndrome

1. Bilateral pyramidal tract signs combined with unilateral or bilateral cranial nerve (III–XI) palsies
2. Vertigo, cerebellar ataxia, visual defects

Internal Carotid Artery Syndrome

1. Most commonly middle cerebral symptoms; also may have parts of anterior and posterior
2. Key sign is monocular blindness on side of occlusion (contralateral to hemiplegia) due to ophthalmic artery involvement

Middle Cerebral Artery Syndrome

(Most commonly occluded) classic stroke syndrome:
1. Contralateral hemiplegia
2. Hemianesthesia
3. Homonymous hemianopsia
4. Global aphasia if dominant hemisphere involved

Posterior Cerebral Artery Syndrome

1. Visual disturbances (line of Genari, layer of occipital, calcarine fissure)
2. Thalamic syndrome
   a. Contralateral hemiparesis and flaccid paralysis
   b. Impairment of deep or superficial sensory system
   c. Agonizing, burning pain
   d. Choreatheosis, alexia and tremor

MISCELLANEOUS VASCULAR TOPICS: KEY WORDS

Anoxic Encephalopathy

1. Can be induced in any patient with insufficient blood supply to brain without a frank infarct
2. Key findings: dropping out of large neurons in
   a. Sommer section of Ammon's horn
   b. Purkinje cells of cerebellum
   c. If severe, laminar necrosis of neurons of cerebral cortex may occur
3. Most common in older patients with severe arteriosclerosis; probably part of senile brain syndrome

Hypertensive Encephalopathy

1. Cerebral edema and/or little infarcts due to hypertension
   Often presents terminally in patients with severe hypertension and renal disease
2. Most common in middle-aged black women
3. Signs and symptoms those of increased intracranial pressure and cerebral edema

Venous Infarcts

1. Due to occlusion of veins draining brain
2. Morphology: small hemorrhagic infarcts in subcortical and cortical regions at *base* of sulci because poorest blood supply is there
3. Most common in children with dehydration

CNS Hemorrhages: Key Words

Type of Hemorrhage	Order of Frequency		Pathology
	Adults	*Infants and Children*	1. Acute: hemorrhage into brain substance and Virchow-Robin spaces
Intracerebral	1. Hypertensive, spontaneous hemorrhage 2. Hemorrhage secondary to thrombi and emboli 3. Overdicumarolization 4. Leukemia: "coin" hemorrhages secondary to leukemic cell aggregates 5. Trauma 6. AV malformations 7. TTP—drug allergy	1. Birth trauma 2. Vitamin K deficiency	2. Chronic: hemosiderin-laden gitter cells in brain substance
Subarachnoid	1. Ruptured berry aneurysm, most common in adults 2. Secondary to trauma 3. Secondary to CVA 4. AV malformations	1. Birth trauma, tearing of great vein of Galen during forceps delivery most common 2. AV malformations 3. Epilepsy with convulsions	1. Diffuse on surface of brain 2. Does not pull off
Subdural	Most commonly due to trauma, with rupture of dural vein Common in old people with mild trauma due to brain atrophy, "pulling dural veins on the stretch"	Trauma	1. Focal collection of blood under dura 2. Goes from black to yellow color with maturation 3. Forms membrane and scar in weeks to months 4. Can cause focal Jacksonian epilepsy
Epidural	Traumatic rupture of middle meningeal artery at foramen spinosum Usually have brief unconsciousness, lucid interval, unconsciousness syndrome	Trauma	1. Blood above dura 2. Patients die if not relieved early, so rarely see chronic healed cases

BERRY ANEURYSMS

Etiology

1. Congenital, almost never seen ruptured in children
2. Absence of media muscle and internal elastic lamina at bifurcation (no external elastic lamina in any intracerebral arteries)

Incidence

Usually occur in 40–60 age group

Location

Order of frequency
1. Middle cerebral artery and branches (29%)
2. Anterior cerebral artery and branches (24.5%)
3. Internal carotid artery (19%)
4. Basilar artery and branches (14.5%)
5. Posterior cerebral artery and branches (6.5%)

Special Features

Multiple in 10%–20% of cases
Size usually 1–3 cm. diameter

Associated Conditions

1. Hypertension
2. Polycystic kidney
3. Postductal coarctation of aorta

Clinical

1. Abrupt onset of severe headache
2. Signs of increased intracranial pressure with unconciousness

Prognosis

Recovery rare with bleeding

CNS TRAUMA

Concussion

1. Loss of consciousness due to sudden blow on head
2. NO morphologic changes associated

Contusion

1. Focal (hemorrhage-infarct-gliosis) lesion of the brain due to sudden trauma
2. Lesion often opposite side of trauma (contra-coup)
3. Sites of predilection (order of frequency):
   a. Tips of temporal lobes
   b. Tips and base of frontal lobes
   c. Tips and base of occipital lobes

Laceration

1. Disruption in continuity of brain substance due to trauma
2. Always get focal hemorrhages and repair, fibrosis (gliosis), yellow scars
3. Scars can be foci for Jacksonian epilepsy

Spinal Cord Injury

Transverse myelitis; most common cause is trauma (hematomyelia)

31 CNS–Tumors

Generalities

Most common malignant tumor IN the CNS is metastatic; the lung is most common primary site
Primary brain tumors rarely metastasize when undisturbed; poor stroma inducers; meningiomas and medulloblastomas can metastasize outside CNS but rarely do

Gliomas			
Astrocytoma	Oligodendroglioma	Ependymoma	Medulloblastoma
Histogenesis			
Astrocytes	Oligodendroglia	Ependymal cells	External (?) granular layer of cerebellar cortex
Incidence			
70–80% of gliomas Most common primary CNS tumor	5% of all gliomas	5% of all gliomas	10% of all gliomas
Clinical			
Most common in middle life Supratentorial in adults; infratentorial in children Gradual onset of symptoms; cerebellar signs and symptoms in children	Most common in young adults	Most common in children and young adults; can occur in adults	Usually in children Cerebellar and midbrain symptoms
Gross			
Homogeneous, yellow, firm, with hemorrhagic areas in high-grade tumor; cysts	Firm, white tumors; hemorrhage rare; calcification seen in about 50% of cases	Most common in 4th ventricle, cysts common; frequent in spinal cord	Always infiltrate from cerebellum, usually in midline

(Continued on overleaf)

Gliomas *(continued)*

Astrocytoma	Oligodendroglioma	Ependymoma	Medulloblastoma

Micro

Astrocytoma	Oligodendroglioma	Ependymoma	Medulloblastoma
Grade I: astrocytes Grade II: astrocytes with pleomorphism Grades III or IV: glioblastoma multiforme 1. Anaplastic astrocytes 2. Endothelial proliferation, necrosis	Excess oligos with perinuclear halo and hyperchromatism Flecks of calcium in over 50% of cases	Low-grade glandular or palisade pattern around cavity (blood vessel) most common Grade IV almost identical to astrocytoma Grade IV Blepharoplasts-tiny rods in cytoplasm between nucleus and lumen (blood vessels)	Small, round cells forming rosettes or pseudorosettes; cells may be carrot shaped

Special Features

Astrocytoma	Oligodendroglioma	Ependymoma	Medulloblastoma
1. Low-grade astrocytoma most common in children and ONLY curable tumor 2. Bipolar cells (spongioblastoma polare) most common tumor in pons in children		1. Second most common adult glioma 2. By EM blepharoplasts are remnants of chromatin granules (centrioles) at base of cilia	Commonly seeds meninges; "frosted" meninges

Prognosis

Astrocytoma	Oligodendroglioma	Ependymoma	Medulloblastoma
1. Average survival: 24–60 mos. 2. Glioblastoma multiforme: 12 mos. 3. Spongioblastoma polare: 46 mos.	Best of gliomas: 5 yrs.	32 mos.	Poor (16 mos.)

Tumors—II

	Meningioma	Neurilemmoma (Schwannoma)	Neurofibroma (Schwannoma)
Histogenesis	Meningothelial cells Fibroblasts	Schwann cells	Schwann cells (?),
Incidence	15% of all intracranial tumors	8% of all intracranial tumors	Common peripherally
Clinical	Variable: symptoms of increased pressure and palsies of nerves, usually in children and young adults	Nerve deafness, tinnitus, vertigo; usually in middle-aged adults	von Recklinghausen's disease of skin and nerves, multiple neurofibromas and cafe-au-lait spots
Location	1. Parasagittal (25%) 2. Floor of anterior fossa (18%) 3. Sphenoid ridge (17%) 4. Convexity of hemispheres (17%) 5. Near sella turcica (8%)	Most common on 8th nerve, cerebellopontine angle 7th nerve 2nd most common, can be seen in any nerve	Usually multiple, commonly on peripheral nerves
Gross	Most are firm, whorled, gray-white Few to several cm. in size Usually solitary	Yellow-white, firm, encapsulated tumor	Small, firm, fibrous tumor; not encapsulated
Micro	3 types (formerly 33) 1. Meningotheliomatous: cluster of cells with fibrous stroma 2. Psammomatous: same as meningotheliomatous, but with psammoma bodies 3. Fibroblastic (least common): elongated fibroblasts, encapsulated	Palisading verocay bodies Antoni A: Palisading cellular areas Antoni B: Acellular cystic areas Reticulum stain positive, may help differentiate it from astrocytoma-low grade	Helter-skelter arrangement of elongated neural cells with hooked nuclei
Special features	1. Cause osteoblastic proliferation of overlying bone 2. Rarely become malignant 3. Can metastasize if malignant but this is very, very rare 4. May be hypoploid 5. Can undergo osseous, cartilaginous, lipid, or other metaplasias	1. Most common tumor of cerebellopontine angle; meningiomas 2nd most common here 2. Do not become malignant (Ackerman) (?) 3. Also seen in mediastinal and peritoneal area	1. Most common primary neoplasm of the spinal cord 2. Have malignant potential, especially if deep; called malignant schwannomas
Prognosis	Good if removed surgically	Good if it can be removed but recurs if not completely removed	Depends on where located and whether benign

Tumors—III

	Pineal Tumors	Colloid Cyst of Third Ventricle
Histogenesis	Pineal cells or cell rests	From choroid plexus cells, paraphysis
Incidence	Less than 1% of brain tumors	Under 2% of intracranial gliomas
Clinical	1. Usually in patients 15–25 yrs. old 2. 88% in males	Most common in 3rd and 4th decade
Symptoms	Due to pressure on 3rd ventricle aqueduct of Sylvius (hydrocephalus)	Acute hydrocephalus, especially with head movement; unexpected death in 20% of cases
Pathology		
Gross	Usually small, white, firm; if large, presses on quadrigeminal plate causing obstruction (hydrocephalus)	Must be over 1 cm. to give symptoms; usually over 2.5 cm. in diameter
Micro	1. Teratomas most common 2. Pinealomas: almost identical to seminomas with lymphocyte stroma 3. Epidermoid inclusion cyst, 4. True gliomas are very rare, look like astrocytomas	Large, single cyst of choroid plexus with cholesterol clefts and foam cells resembling plaque; lined with cuboidal epithelial cells with cilia or apocrine type cells
Special comment	1. Tumor may cause precocious or delayed puberty 2. Melatonin inhibits MSH, Interferes with skin pigmentation 3. "Seat of the soul"	No symptoms unless occlude 3rd ventricle
Prognosis	Good if can be removed surgically	Excellent with removal

"APUDOMAS" AND THE APUD "SYSTEM"

Introduction

Recently, lesions involving cells with "A" high amine content, "P" precursor (DOPA or 5 HTP), "U" uptake and "D" high decarboxylase activity have been grouped together and called the "APUD system." These cells are said to be of neuroectoderm or neural crest origin. These cells secrete either polypeptides or amine hormones or both. Anatomically, these cells are quite diffuse in the body, being generally characterized as:

1. Central (hypothalamic, pineal, etc.)
2. Alimentary (pancreas, especially islet of Langerhans, stomach and intestine)
3. General (thyroid "C" cells, lungs—Kulchitsky cells—"P" cells and adrenal medulla and skin melanocytes)

General Characteristics of APUD Cells (besides those named above):

1. Ultrastructurally, they contain endocrine granules oriented toward vascular pole of the cells
2. Specific immunofluorescence
3. High peroxidase activity

Comments

1. While the APUD concept is an interesting one linking these cells embryologically, structurally, and physiologically, its usefulness in the management of such diffuse diseases of the system "APUDOMAS" ranging from insulinoma to malignant melanoma has yet to be demonstrated
2. Possibly with further investigation, the use of "specific drugs" affecting various parts of the "APUD" system may become useful in clinical medicine

32 CNS–Infectious Diseases

Meningitis—I

	Pyogenic	*Tuberculous*
Etiology	Order of frequency in U.S.A. 1. Pneumococcus (adults) 2. Meningococcus (epidemics) 3. *H. influenzae* (most common in children) 4. Often part of generalized septicemia	*M. tuberculosis* usually secondary to miliary pulmonary TBC
Clinical features	1. Headache, photophobia 2. Stiff neck, meningeal irritation 3. Kernig's sign (pain on leg extension) 4. Later coma	Slower in onset but symptoms same as pyogenic meningitis
CSF	High-protein, high cells, low sugar, low chloride, positive culture	High protein, low sugar and chloride; pellicle in CSF on standing
Gross	Thickened meninges and pus, usually along blood vessels Pneumococcus over convexity of brain Meningococcus and *H. influenzae* at base of brain	Thick meninges at base of brain and spinal cord
Micro	Polys, edema, early; organization late	Langhans' giant cells, granulomata, also ependymitis granularis
Special features	1. May occlude foramina of Luschka and Magendie, internal hydrocephalus 2. Nerve palsy occurs 3. Waterhouse-Friderichsen in 20% of meningococcal cases 4. May get subdural empyema (abscess)	1. May heal with chronic granulomata 2. Probably most common cause of occluded Luschka-Magendie (Dandy's syndrome) 3. 20% mortality with treatment 4. 100% mortality without treatment

Meningitis—II

	Fungal	Viral
Etiology	Cryptococcosis (torulosis) most common fungal cause of meningitis, and the most common cause of chronic meningitis	Lymphocytic choriomeningitis (LCM) virus, most commonly from MICE
Clinical	Similar to TB Usually also have pulmonary cryptococcosis	Grippelike syndrome with stiff neck, spontaneous recovery in 7–10 days Leukopenia common
CSF	India-ink preparation for diagnosis	1. Up to 30,000 lymphocytes/cu. mm. 2. Increased CSF pressure 3. No bacteria, can culture virus from CSF
Gross	Basal, fibrinopurulent, shaggy exudate	Slight thickening and hypermia of meninges
Micro	Lymphocytes, monocytes, organisms, cysts in depths of sulci	Lymphocytes in meninges
Special features	1. Patients often have other debilitating disease, especially lymphomas and leukemias 2. Commonly associated with pulmonary TBC	1. Aseptic meningitis, no bacteria or fungi 2. Usually associated with viral infection

BRAIN ABSCESS

Etiology

1. Direct route: 40% of all brain abscesses from mastoiditis (tegmen tympani most common site for invasion); 10% of all brain abscesses from frontal sinuses; trauma an uncommon cause
2. Hematogenous route: most common from suppurative pneumonic process; common with congenital heart disease, especially with right-to-left shunt; also common with SBE and septicemia

Bacteria

Streptococci, pneumococci, staphylococci, and gram-negatives

Gross

1. Edema: flat gyri, narrow sulci, uncal herniation, cingulate gyrus herniation
2. Pus-filled cavity, fibrous capsule
3. Usually singular

Micro

1. Polys: necrosis, bacteria, (inner layer)
2. *Fibrosis:* fibroblasts (capsule)
3. Gliosis: gitter cells, gemistocytic astrocytes in surrounding brain
4. Edema: swollen oligodendroglia in surrounding brain

Prognosis

1. Without treatment, nearly 100% mortality
2. With treatment, 40% mortality
3. Very rare for them to heal spontaneously

PROTOZOAL DISEASES: KEY WORDS

Toxoplasmosis

1. Granulomatous meningitis and encephalitis
2. Focal calcification of brain
3. Also calcification in lungs, RE system and striated muscle
4. Mental deficiency and convulsions
5. Most commonly acquired in utero

Trypanosomiasis (Sleeping Sickness)

1. Gambesian and Rhodesian types
2. Tsetse fly is insect vector
3. Morular cells in glial reaction
4. Mortality: Rhodesian 100% (no chronic stage)
        Gambesian 50%

Metazoal Disease (Cysticercosis Cellulosae)

1. Due to *T. solium (Cysticercus cellulosae)* larvae
2. Encystment with inflammation
3. Causes 10% of Jacksonian seizures in Mexico

Neurosyphilis

	Meningovascular	*Tabes Dorsalis*	*General Paresis*
Clinical	1. Increased intracranial pressure 2. Cranial nerve palsy 3. Focal cerebral signs and symptoms, often of sudden onset 4. Paresthesias, weakness, sensory loss in extremities (spinal cord)	1. Lightning-like pains in legs and abdomen 2. Argyll Robertson pupil (no reaction to light, but reaction to accommodation) 3. Loss of deep tendon reflexes 4. Impairment of proprioception 5. Charcot joints (painless, swollen); most common cause of Charcot joint in lower extremity	1. Personality changes 2. COBS (chronic organic brain syndrome) 3. Mental deterioration

(Continued on facing page)

Neurosyphilis *(continued)*

	Meningovascular	Tabes Dorsalis	General Paresis
Pathology	1. Leptomeningitis: base with nerve palsies and CSF obstruction 2. Hydrocephalus 3. Arteritis, perivascular lymphocytes and plasma cells 4. Degeneration of nerve roots 5. Gummas, focal granulomas of meninges can occur	1. Leptomeningitis 2. Degeneration of posterior roots and dorsal funiculus	1. Meningoencephalitis 2. Brain atrophy 3. Ependymitis granularis 4. Disorganized architecture; Key word: windswept cortex 5. Rod cells phagocytize spirochetes and iron
Special features		Optic atrophy in 10%	

Viruses of the Nervous System—I

	Poliomyelitis	Rabies
Virus	Polio virus, 3 types	Rabies virus
Clinical	Usually in children	Any age
	Acute febrile illness early Flaccid paralysis later	History of dog bite, convulsions, salivation (hydrophobia); incubation period depends on distance of bite from CNS
Gross	Congestion, focal hemorrhage in cord and medulla	Cerebral edema and focal hemorrhage
Micro	Early: neutrophils Late: loss of anterior horn cells and gliosis, neuronophagia (oligodendroglia)	Negri bodies in cytoplasm of Purkinje cells and large neurons of Sommer sector (Ammon's horn) of hippocampus
Special features	1. Rare now, due to vaccine 2. Only 6000 cases per year at peak incidence	1. Must quarantine dogs 10 days; if no symptoms, OK 2. If dog has symptoms, kill and look for Negri bodies; if positive, give vaccine 3. Encephalomyelitis is a danger of vaccine; vaccination is also painful 4. Less danger now with duck embryo vaccine

VIRUSES OF THE NERVOUS SYSTEM—II: KEY WORDS

Equine Encephalitis

Western:
1. Horses, mosquitoes
2. Neutrophils in CSF early, mononuclear cells later
3. 10% mortality (prognosis better than EEE)

Eastern:
1. Horses, mosquitoes
2. Neutrophils, then monocytes in CSF
3. 50%–75% mortality (prognosis worse than WEE)

Japanese B Encephalitis

1. Mosquito is vector
2. Usually recover completely
3. Involves basal nuclei, floor of 4th ventricle and cerebral and cerebellar gray matter

Postvaccinal Encephalitis

1. 1/100,000 smallpox vaccinations
2. If survive, sequelae rare
3. 40% mortality

Herpes Zoster

1. Same virus as varicella
2. Has distribution of one dorsal nerve
3. Inflammatory reaction in dorsal nerve root cells
4. Commonly associated with lymphomas and leukemia
5. Can have meningitis or encephalitis

Herpes Simplex

1. Herpes simplex virus
2. Predilection for medial, basal part of temporal lobes and the insula
3. Very destructive
4. Can use FA to identify on biopsies

Secondary Postinfectious Encephalomyelitis

1. Can get encephalitis after almost any viral infection (e.g., measles, chickenpox, mumps, etc.)
2. Probably due to autoimmune response
3. Demyelination and inflammatory cell reaction; early—polys; later—chronic inflammatory cells

	von Economo Encephalitis (Encephalitis Lethargica) vs.	St. Louis Encephalitis
Virus	Not isolated	Virus isolated
Clinical	Young adults, high fever with CNS symptoms Coma, rigidity, etc.	A variety of von Economo encephalitis (?)
Gross	Congestion and focal hemorrhage	Congestion and focal hemorrhage
Micro	Perivascular cuffing in CNS, degeneration of nerve cells	Perivascular cuffing in CNS, degeneration of nerve cells, neutrophils in meninges
Special features	1. Parkinson's disease, common in people who were young adults in 1918–1926 2. Parkinson's disease incidence decreasing now	1. Residua severe 2. No cases of true parkinsonism associated 3. Culex mosquito is vector, but horses are not reservoir

"Slow" Virus Diseases of the CNS

	Kuru (K)	Jakob-Creutzfeldt (J-C)	Subacute Sclerosing Panencephalitis (SSPE)	Progressive Multifocal Leukoencephalopathy (PML)
Clinical	Exotic, subacute, progressive CNS disease of New Guinea natives who practice cannibalism: ataxia, tremors, dysarthria Fatal in 3–9 months	Myoclonus, fasciculation, spasticity, dementia ataxia Usually in late middle age Patients usually die in a few months	Slow-wave EEG changes, paretic colloidal gold curve, mostly in children under 10 years; progressive myoclonic jerking, afebrile with motor disability Fatal in 1–3 years	In patients with carcinoma, Hodgkin's, sarcoid, TBC, leukemia, lymphoma, etc.
Virus	Not yet identified	Not yet identified	Measles virus	Papovavirus
Pathology	Degenerative spongiform encephalopathy with intranuclear vacuolization of neurons	Identical to kuru with amyloid-containing plaques of Alzheimer type Loss of neurons without significant inflammation Chronic histology with acute course	Measles virus antibody found in cells, tubular structures in intranuclear inclusions on EM; degeneration of neurons	EM intranuclear crystalline mass = Papovavirus

(Continued on overleaf)

"Slow" Virus Diseases of the CNS *(continued)*

	Kuru (K)	Jakob-Creutzfeldt (J-C)	Subacute Sclerosing Panencephalitis (SSPE)	Progressive Multifocal Leukoencephalo-pathy (PML)
Special	Has been passed to monkey brains	1. Has been passed to monkeys 2. Incubation period: 11–14 months 3. Scrapie and mink encephalopathy have very similar findings 4. Spongiform encephalopathy probably a variant	1. Incubation period of a few months to 10 years 2. Viron not present in fully synchronous form 3. NOT same as postmeasles encephalitis 4. High measles antibody titer; (?) hypersensitivity disease	1. Virus cannot be distinguished from polyoma or SV 40 virus 2. Probably due to activation of latent virus due to immunosup-pression

33 CNS–Degeneration and Miscellaneous Topics

Degeneration of CNS—I

	Alzheimer's Disease (Presenile Atrophy)	Pick's Disease (Lobar Atrophy)	Senile Brain (Senile Dementia)
Etiology	AUTOSOMAL DOMINANT IN SOME CASES		Arteriosclerosis (?) Aging (?)
Clinical	1. Progressive 2. Presenile (40's–50's) dementia and disturbance in speech 3. About 10% have convulsions 4. NO cranial nerve palsy; hemiplegia or hemianesthesia	1. Symptoms less severe than Alzheimer's, but often cannot differentiate clinically 2. Affects more women than men	1. Dementia progressive in old-age group (65+) 2. COBS (most common cause of) 3. May or may not have strokes
Gross	*Diffuse* symmetric atrophy of cerebral cortex	Extreme "knife-blade" atrophy of frontal and temporal lobes, often asymmetric	1. Small, firm brain 2. Atrophy of gyri, especially frontal lobe 3. Calcified arachnoidal villi
Micro	1. Neurofibrillary (tangles) degeneration marked 2. Argentophile plaques (Alzheimer's plaques) may be same as senile plaques	1. Argentophilic degeneration of neurons with gliosis 2. Ballooned neurons 3. No neurofibrillary tangles or senile plaques	1. Decreased neurons, increased glia 2. Senile plaques, best seen with silver stain, only in gray matter (dead neuron with dendritic processes and amyloid) 3. Neurofibrillary changes, less common, seen more in Alzheimer's (neurofibrils tangled within neuron)

(Continued on overleaf)

Degeneration of CNS—I *(continued)*

	Alzheimer's Disease (Presenile Atrophy)	Pick's Disease (Lobar Atrophy)	Senile Brain (Senile Dementia)
EM	*Neurofibrillary degeneration:* twisted tubules from normal neuronal microtubules		*Senile plaques:* degenerating dendritic aggregates with lysosomes and mitochondria, often twisted tubules (late: extracellular amyloid)
Special features	1. Both are rare diseases almost equally frequent 2. Distinguished from senile dementia by age of patient and lack of arteriosclerosis		Poor correlation between amount of gross and micro changes and symptoms

Degeneration of CNS-II

	Parkinson's Disease	Amyotrophic Lateral Sclerosis	Progressive Muscular Atrophy
Etiology	1. Postencephalitic: history, oily skin, EOM palsies 2. Cerebrovascular: sudden steplike onset 3. Idiopathic: most common now	Unknown, some cases autosomal dominant Hereditary; environment (?) 15% of Guamanians die of ALS No increase in military personnel on Guam	Unknown Hereditary (?)
Clinical	1. Pill-rolling tremor 2. Cogwheel rigidity 3. Stumbling gait 4. Masklike face	1. Middle-age group peak 2. Fasciculation of muscles 3. Begins in small muscles of hands	1. Several syndromes 2. Marie-Charcot-Tooth peroneal muscular atrophy, most common
Gross	Pigment loss in substantia nigra, locus ceruleus and red nucleus (most severe in postencephalitic)	Muscle atrophy pattern	Muscle atrophy pattern in affected groups
Micro	1. Intracellular eosinophilic bodies (Lewy bodies— lysosomes) in neurons of substantia nigra of idiopathic cases (84%); of postencephalitic cases (44%) 2. Loss of neurons and variable atrophy and gliosis in basal ganglia	1. Degeneration of BOTH upper (Betz) and lower (anterior horn cells) motor neurons 2. Late: degeneration pons and medulla	1. Degeneration of anterior horn cells 2. Degeneration of axis cylinders

(Continued on facing page)

Degeneration of CNS—II *(continued)*

	Parkinson's Disease	Amyotrophic Lateral Sclerosis	Progressive Muscular Atrophy
Special features	1. Parkinson's peak age increasing more rapidly than general population age 2. No slow virus yet! 3. Increased iron in brain 4. Can get parkinsonlike syndrome with drugs (e.g., reserpine and phenothiazines)	1. Progressive bulbar palsy is a variant 2. Infantile muscular atrophy (Werdnig-Hoffmann syndrome), rare hereditary in infants, anterior horn cells and medulla atrophy	1. Other "fancy" neurologic syndromes 2. May be a variant of ALS

Demyelinating Diseases—I

	Multiple Sclerosis (MS)	Schilder's Disease (Diffuse Sclerosis)
Etiology	Unknown, autoimmune (?), animal experiments; *degeneration of oligodendroglia,* often precipitated by fever, trauma, stress, slow virus (?)	Unknown
Clinical	Uncommon, age 20–40 years usually; multiple neurologic symptoms with remission and exacerbation, blindness, paresthesias, etc.; Charcot's triad: nystagmus, intention tremor, staccato speech	Rare, most common under 12 yrs. of age; variable, but progressive, blindness, spastic paralysis and mental failure are the usual sequence
Gross	Multiple, small, gray, translucent patches in white matter, especially in pons, medulla, and cerebellar peduncles	Marked, diffuse demyelinization of cerebral hemispheres and brain stem; U fibers spared
Micro	Early: fragmented myelin, few lymphocytes and plasma cells, axons preserved, then late: glial scars (gliosis)	Early: (lipid-laden phagocytes) lymphocytes and plasma cells. Late: gliosis (similar to multiple sclerosis)
Special features	1. Neuromyelitis optica, predominantly eye involvement with transverse myelitis 2. Prognosis variable few months to several years 3. MS the most common cause of demyelinization in the U.S.A. 4. Early remissions because of preservation of axons even with myelin degeneration 5. Increased incidence with HLA-A7, HLA-B18, and LD-7a; (?) hereditary	1. Swayback in lambs, similar gross and micro, due to copper deficiency 2. Prognosis: usually fatal in 1–3 years

DEMYELINATING DISEASES: KEY WORDS

Krabbes Leukodystrophy

Lipid-filled foreign body giant cells in lesions; basic defect-beta-galactocerebrosidase deficiency with ceramide galactoside being stored

Metachromatic Leukodystrophy

Metachromatic material in neuronal cells of brain, spinal cord; Kupffer cells of liver; renal tubular cells; basic defect-arylsulfatase A deficiency, store acid sphingoglycolipid; poor phagocytosis of lipids in brain

Pelizaeus-Merzbacher Disease (Glycerolphosphatide Dystrophy)

Familial, very rare; protracted course, pyramidal and extrapyramidal signs without blindness; preservation of small islands of myelin around blood vessels in areas of demyelination
Etiology: (?) failure of myelin development or degeneration

COMMON METABOLIC DISEASES OF NERVOUS SYSTEM: KEY WORDS

Hepatic Encephalopathy

High blood ammonia; hypertrophy and hyperplasia of protoplasmic astrocytes (also seen in uremia)

Tay-Sachs Disease (Amaurotic Familial Idiocy)

Ganglioside GM-2 in lysosomes of nerve cells; enzymatic defects; (hexosamidase A in garden variety); both A and B absent in variant and beta galactosidases A, B, C absent in generalized gangliosidosis; cherry-red spot in macula

Wilson's Disease (Hepatolenticular Degeneration)

Hereditary; Kayser-Fleischer rings in Descemet's membrane of cornea; degeneration of corpus striatum (basal ganglia); cirrhosis, portal type; increased copper in tissue; decreased serum copper and ceruloplasmin

SOME COMMON NUTRITIONAL DISEASES OF NERVOUS SYSTEM: KEY WORDS

Korsakoff's Psychosis (Dementia)

Thiamine deficiency; confabulation, memory loss; bilateral atrophy and orange pigmentation of mamillary bodies; may be a part of Wernicke's encephalopathy

Subacute Combined Systems Disease

Due to vitamin B_{12} deficiency; NOT treated with folic acid (made worse by folic acid); involves crossed and uncrossed pyramidal tracts, and posterior columns

Wernicke's Encephalopathy (paralysis of eye muscles, confusion, stupor, death)

Thiamine deficiency; common in alcoholics; hemorrhage and gliosis in mamillary bodies; also may involve periventricular nuclei; also may have symptoms of heart disease (beriberi)

COMMON CNS POISONS: KEY WORDS

Carbon Monoxide Poisoning

ACUTE: cherry-red livor mortis; bilateral basal ganglion necrosis;

CHRONIC: bilaterial basal ganglion necrosis, often with calcification

Acute Lead Poisoning

Mostly children, cerebral edema; focal petechial hemorrhages due to anoxia

Methyl Alcohol Poisoning

Blindness due to degeneration of ganglion cells of retina; no other *specific* nerve cell changes

Ethyl Alcohol Ingestion

Characteristic but not necessarily diagnostic nervous system effects include:
1. Wernicke's encephalopathy and Korsakoff's psychosis (see above)
2. Central pontine myelinolysis
3. Cerebellar atrophy, especially in the vermes
4. Excess proliferation of protoplasmic astrocytes
5. Alzheimer's Type II astrocytes: associated with cirrhosis, secondary to alcoholism
6. Contusions, multiple, especially in temporal, occipital, and frontal tips and base of frontal lobes
7. Peripheral neuropathy may occur, especially with thiamine and niacin deficiency

"UNUSUAL" NEUROLOGIC DISEASES: KEY WORDS

Friedreich's Ataxia (Ataxia Pes Cavus Kyphoscoliosis)

1. Hereditary
2. Begins in childhood
3. Involves posterior and lateral columns
4. Cerebellar reel: cerebellar tracts
5. Commonly have myocarditis with degeneration and vacuolation of myocardial cells

Huntington's Chorea

1. Dominant heredity
2. Bilateral degeneration of caudate nucleus in adult life, symptoms begin in adult life

Spongiform Encephalopathy

1. Slow virus
2. Spongy brain
3. Similar to Jakob-Creutzfeldt

Syringomyelia (Cyst Syrinx [Tube] in Spinal Cord)

1. Etiology unknown: 75% are low grade astrocytomas, 25% classic cysts
2. MOST common in lower cervical cord, SECOND most common in lumbar cord
3. Anesthesia of arms: most common cause of Charcot's joint of elbow
4. Cyst NOT lined with ependyma
5. Gliosis precedes cyst formation

Tuberous Sclerosis

1. Autosomal dominant heredity
2. Syndrome: mental retardation and sebaceous adenomas of skin
3. "Candle dripping" on ventricular surfaces of brain (gliosis with calcification)
4. Commonly associated with visceral tumors and cysts, especially rhabdomyosarcomas and cysts of the pancreas

Reye's Syndrome

1. Etiology obscure, but mostly seen after viral infection; influenza B virus most common
2. Syndrome includes lowered levels of blood glucose, arginine, and citrulline; high levels of ammonia, glutamine, alanine and lysine, mostly in children
3. Fatty degeneration of visceral organs, especially liver
4. CNS: degeneration of pyramidal cells, metabolic changes with Type II astrocytes and edema

Guillain-Barre Syndrome vs. Landry's Paralysis

	Guillain-Barre	Landry's
Clinical	Both syndromes nearly identical except Guillain-Barre patients tend to have more severe illness	
Symptoms	Infectious polyneuritis; 2/3 have history of (12 days) previous URI, paralysis of cranial nerves (7th and 10th most common)	
	Facial diplegia (85%) Dysphagia or dysarthria (50%) 11th nerve weakness (20%)	
	Eye muscle rarely involved, muscle tenderness is moderate, fever is common, more severe in Guillain-Barre	
Albumino-cytological disassociation	Yes	No
CSF findings	CSF protein commonly over 1000 mg.% CSF cells 10–100	CSF protein under 100 mg.% CSF cells 10–100
Pathology	Neurons of medulla and spinal cord show retrograde (axonal) degeneration; no inflammatory change in PNS or CNS	No significant change or slight round cell infiltration in spinal ganglia
Mortality rate	6%–60% various series	Under 10%

——————————————— CORTISONE HELPS BOTH ———————

Special comments	1. Either may be mistaken for poliomyelitis. 2. Guillain-Barre may occur after influenza vaccination, especially A New Jersey 876. 3. Some authors consider Guillain-Barre and Landry's as a single syndrome. 4. Albuminocytologic disassociation also seen in diphtheric polyneuritis, diabetic polyneuritis, and occasionally, poliomyelitis after second week.

34 Eye and Ear

KEY OPHTHALMOLOGIC GLOSSARY

Amblyopia

Decreased vision from any cause, without significant objective clinical or ocular abnormality

Ametropia

Ocular refractive error in which the image is not properly focused on the retina; major subtypes are:
Astigmatism: characterized by variations in refraction in the different ocular meridians
Hyperopia (farsightedness): image is focused behind retina
Myopia (nearsightedness): image is focused in front of retina
Presbyopia: characterized by loss of power of accommodation due to lenticular changes associated with aging

Angioid Streaks

Irregular, red-brown bands radiating outward around optic disk and due to degenerative changes and defects in Bruch's membrane (inner choroid); this finding frequently associated with macular degeneration and hemorrhage or with pseudoxanthoma elasticum, and occasionally with Paget's disease of bone; also in sickle cell disease and trait

Blepharitis

Inflammation of eyelid margin

Blindness

Inability to see better than 20/200 with corrective glasses (IRS definition).
Most common causes: children—iridocyclitis secondary to JRA; adults—diabetic retinopathy

Cotton-Wool Spots

Fluffy, white spots in retina and optic disk due to presence of cytoid bodies and serous transudate in layer of nerve fibers, (blocked axoplasmic flow (?), these are nonspecific findings but commonly occur in cases of hypertensive retinopathy, papilledema, occulsion of central retinal vein, lupus erythematosus, and dermatomyositis

Dacryocystitis

Inflammation of lacrimal sac

Ectropion

Eversion of eyelid

Iris Bombé

Anterior bulging of iris due to increased aqueous pressure in posterior chamber; this condition results from pupillary aqueous blockage, as by adhesion of the pupillary margin of the iris to anterior surface of lens (annular posterior synechiae) resulting from iritis

Keratitic Precipitates (KP)

Focal accumulations of cells of an inflammatory exudate and proliferating corneal endothelium on posterior surface of the cornea; secondary to chronic intraocular inflammation

Keratomalacia

Retrogressive softening of cornea; may be due to vitamin A deficiency

Papilledema

Swelling of optic disk (disk elevated more than seven diopters from optic cup); usually due to edema (implies increased intracranial pressure) although hyperemia, hemorrhage, and exudate in disk may be factors

Synechia

Adhesion of iris to an adjacent structure
Anterior synechia: adhesion of iris to inner surface of trabecular meshwork or cornea
Anterior peripheral synechia: adhesion of anterior peripheral iridic surface to inner surface of trabecular meshwork and peripheral cornea
Posterior synechia: adhesion between posterior iridic surface and anterior lenticular surface
Annular posterior synechia: adhesion of entire pupillary margin to lens; synechias are most often secondary to intraocular inflammation, particularly anterior uveitis; they tend to block aqueous outflow

Uveitis

Inflammation of uveal tract
Anterior uveitis: inflammation of iris and ciliary body
Posterior uveitis: inflammation of choroid

Xerophthalmia (Xerosis)

Abnormal dryness of conjunctival sac due to inadequate lacrimal secretion, often due to vitamin A deficiency

ANATOMY REVIEW

(From Duke-Elder)

General

1. Anterior chamber (aqueous)
2. Posterior chamber (aqueous)
3. Vitreous (behind lens)

Tunica Fibrosa

1. Sclera—posterior 5/6ths, by linear measure (white of eye)
   3 layers:
   a. Episclera
   b. Sclera
   c. Lamina fusca (vascular layer)

2. Cornea, anterior 1/6th by linear measure (clear transparent front of eyeball)
   5 layers:
   a. Corneal epithelium
   b. Anterior elastic layer (Bowman's membrane)
   c. Substantia propria
   d. Posterior elastic layer (Descemet's membrane—collagen ?)
   e. Endothelium of anterior chamber

Vascular Coat (Uveal Tract)

1. Choroid: from vitreous chamber to ora serrata
2. Ciliary body: contracts lens and focuses vision, extends from ora serrata to anterior portion of vitreous chamber
3. Iris
   Color of eyes
   Iris angle; spaces of Fontana, canal of Schlemm

Lens

Focus, vision

Retina (10 Layers)

Rods, cones, ganglion cells
Special areas:
   Macula lutea
   Fovea centralis, most cones (precision vision)

Optic Nerve Head

Elevated in papilledema
Excavated in glaucoma
Dura and pia mater are sheaths

DISEASES OF THE EYE

Retrogressive Diseases of the Cornea

CORNEAL DYSTROPHIES: KEY WORDS

Epithelial

1. *Keratoconjunctivitis sicca:* part of Sjogren's syndrome (enlarged parotid glands, lacrimal glands, hyposecretion and keratoconjunctivitis sicca)
2. *Keratomalacia:* vitamin A deficiency
   a. Mucous epithelium to squamous type (squamous metaplasia)
   b. Vascularization may occur
3. *Fuchs' corneal dystrophy:* endothelial and epithelial dystrophy (i.e., Fuchs' dystrophy)

Stromal

Bowman's membrane does not extend to edge of cornea, so have clear zone at periphery when deposit is in Bowman's membrane
1. *Band keratopathy*
   a. Secondary to primary eye disease or hypercalcemia, hyperparathyroidism, sarcoidosis
   b. Begins at edge of Bowman's membrane and spreads centrally

2. *Arcus senilis*
   a. Lipid deposits in stroma
   b. A sign of hyperlipidemia and/or arteriosclerosis
3. *Hurler's disease*
   Gargoylism
   Mucopolysaccharides in stroma

   Gargoylism
   Mucopolysaccharides in stroma

Endothelial

1. *Cornea guttata:* central endothelial dystrophy of cornea
   a. Irregular, warty, diffuse, central thickening of Descemet's membrane
   b. Degenerative changes of endothelium
   c. More common in females than males
   d. Commonly precedes Fuchs' epithelial dystrophy (loss of sensation, superficial central corneal cloudiness)
   e. Leads to overhydration of cornea, epithelial edema and bullae
2. *Hassal-Henle warts*
   a. Warty thickening of Descemet's membrane similar to cornea guttata EXCEPT peripheral in location
   b. Not associated with epithelial edema
   c. Common in eyes after age 40
3. *Kayser-Fleischer rings*
   a. Wilson's disease
   b. Red-green band of copper
   c. Located in posterior half of Descemet's membrane

GLAUCOMA: KEY WORDS

1. Common disease (second most common cause of adult onset blindness in U.S.A.)
2. Definition: increased pressure in eye, usually due to poor drainage of aqueous humor due to any cause
3. Can cause blindness
4. Several types:
   a. *Primary wide angle:* commonest, usually in people over 40 years, bilateral and familial, etiology unknown
   b. *Primary narrow angle:* adults with hyperopia; etiology—shallow anterior filtration angle
   c. *Congenital glaucoma:* present at birth, rare
   d. *Secondary glaucoma:* secondary to other eye diseases (almost any other eye disease can cause it)

DISEASES OF THE LENS: KEY WORDS

Cataract—Opacification of the Lens

1. Senile, most common type of cataract
2. Other types:
   a. Congenital (11 types of congenital cataracts are currently recognized)
   b. Traumatic
   c. Metabolic
      Diabetes most common cause (sorbitol), excess steroids can cause

DISEASES OF THE RETINA: KEY WORDS

Retinitis Pigmentosa

1. Hereditary: order of frequency, autosomal recessive, autosomal dominant, sex-linked recessive
2. Onset—ages 6–13 years, more common in males than females
3. Progressive degeneration of rods first, then cones
4. Phagocytes hold pigment, blindness

Retrolental Fibroplasia

1. Bilateral in infants
2. Due to excess oxygen therapy—iatrogenic—(usually over 40%)
3. Fibrosis and scarring of retina, and vitreous (white reflex), blindness

Hypertensive Retinopathy

1. AV nicking
2. Copper wire, silver wire changes
3. Cotton-wool patches
4. Hemorrhages, exudates and papilledema

Diabetic Retinopathy

1. Capillary microaneurysms, sheathing, vascular proliferation (proliferative retinopathy), hemorrhages and exudates
2. Usually also have diabetic nephropathy
3. Key words: diabetes MOST common cause of acquired blindness in U.S.A. today

Retinal Detachment

Most common cause in U.S.A.—Children: trauma; adults: postcataract extraction. Also may occur with diabetes, trauma, or congenitally

Sympathetic Ophthalmia

1. Granulomatous uveitis due to hypersensitivity reaction; auto-antibodies to injured uveal tissue
2. Follows penetrating ocular injuries
3. Nonnecrotizing granulomatous uveitis in (exciting) eye
4. Two weeks to 1 year, get granulomatous uveitis in other (sympathizing) eye
5. Blindness results
6. Enucleation of exciting eye before 10 days of injury prevents disease

RARE BENIGN INTRAOCULAR TUMORS

Hemangiomas as part of:
1. Sturge-Weber disease (see Chap. 10)—choroidal
2. von Hippel-Lindau disease (see Chap. 10)—retinal

RARE MALIGNANT INTRAOCULAR TUMORS

Melanoma

1. Most common primary malignant intraocular tumor in adults
2. Arises in choroid (usually)
3. Rare in children
4. Rare in blacks

Retinoblastoma

1. Most common primary malignant intraocular tumor in children (white reflex)
2. Rare after 10 years of age
3. 75% occur before 3 years of age
4. Hereditary: occurs in 50% of offspring of patients with retinoblastoma; 33% are bilateral
5. Micro looks identical to neuroblastoma, Ewing's tumor, and medulloblastoma (small, round lymphocytelike cells with rosettes and pseudorosettes)
6. 85% 5-year survival

DISEASES OF THE SCLERA: KEY WORDS

Blue Sclera

1. Due to generalized abnormal mesenchymal development
2. Osteogenesis imperfecta
   a. Brittle bones
   b. Blue sclera
   c. Deafness also common

Sparganosis

1. Use of meat as poultice on a black eye
2. Tapeworm infection in eye
3. Common in Orient, rare in U.S.A.

MISCELLANEOUS DISEASES OF THE EYE: KEY WORDS

Conjunctivitis

1. Most common disease of the eye
2. Ophthalmia neonatorum: *N. gonorrhoeae*
3. Pink eye: *H. aegyptius* (Koch-Weeks bacillus)
4. Trachoma virus: keratoconjunctivitis is the most common cause of blindness in Southeast Asia and other endemic areas; rare in U.S.A.
5. Inclusion blenorrhea: promiscuous adults

Hordeolum (Sty)

1. Folliculitis of eyelid
2. Most commonly due to staphylococcus

Chalazion

Chronic lipogranulomas in Meibomian or Zeis glands due to retained lipid in glandular secretions

Xanthelasma

Yellow lesion, usually in skin of medial eyelid; lipid-laden macrophages, associated with high blood lipid and arteriosclerosis

Pinguecula

1. Yellow tinted nodules, bulbar conjunctiva in old age and in Gaucher's disease
2. Senile elastosis and hyperplasia of conjunctival stroma
3. Cosmetic problem only

Phlyctenular Keratoconjunctivitis

1. Allergy to *M. tuberculosis; S. aureus*
2. Usually in children
3. Key symptom—photophobia

DISEASES OF THE EAR: SPECIAL TOPICS

Cholesteatoma

1. Proliferation of stratified squamous epithelial cells; a variant of epidermal inclusion cyst. Cholesterol crystals only occur with degeneration
2. Most common location in otic canal and mastoid areas
3. Importance:
   Enlarge and erode bones
   Prevent healing of mastoiditis and otitis
   May cause meningitis by bone erosion
4. Only treatment is surgery

Labyrinthitis

Most commonly due to otitis media

Mastoiditis

1. Usually secondary to otitis
2. Acute, most commonly due to beta hemolytic streptococcus
   Complications: osteomyelitis, meningitis
   Bezold's abscess: posterior cervical abscess is a complication
3. Chronic: fibrosis and cholesteatoma

Meniere's Disease

1. Syndrome: tinnitus, deafness and vertigo
2. Hydrops of labyrinth, dilatation of cochlear duct, saccule, utricle, and increased endolymphatic lymph
3. Onset usually after 30 years of age and usually unilateral
4. No perfect treatment

Neurolabyrinthine Disease

1. Bacterial endotoxins
2. Quinine, salicylates
   Streptomycin (dizziness)
   Dihydrostreptomycin (deafness)
   Neomycin, kanamycin, ethacrynic acid
   Gentamycin (damage to vestibular apparatus)
3. Excess noise, degeneration of organ of Corti, deafness

Otitis Media

1. Most commonly (66%) due to bacteria
2. Acute: most common in children; *Streptococcus pneumoniae* is the most common cause
3. Recurrent: variety of bacteria, staph and *H. influenzae*
4. Chronic otitis may be a continuation of acute, gram-negative bacteria and mixed bacteria are frequent

5. Complications: brain abscess, especially in temporal lobe, meningitis, jugular phlebitis; added complications of chronic otitis include sclerosis, scarring, and cholesteatoma
6. Serous otitis: clear eardrum
   Etiology unknown, may lead to deafness and sclerosis

Otosclerosis

1. Deafness due to ossification and bony ankylosis of footplate of stapes in the oval window, usually bilateral
2. Etiology unknown, hereditary (?)
3. A very common cause of conductive deafness
4. Most frequent in 12–35-year-old white females, onset frequently with menarche or pregnancy
5. Uncommon in blacks
6. Need surgery to treat

Presbycusis (Senile Deafness)

1. Onset in old age common
2. Perceptive high-tone deafness
3. Atrophy of spiral ganglion in *basal* turn of cochlea

Index